Standing at
Water's Edge

Standing at Water's Edge

A Cancer Nurse,
Her Four-Year-Old Son
and the Shifting Tides of Leukemia

JANICE POST-WHITE

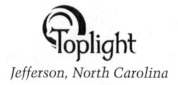

Jefferson, North Carolina

ISBN (print) 978-1-4766-8710-0
ISBN (ebook) 978-1-4766-4464-6

LIBRARY OF CONGRESS AND BRITISH LIBRARY
CATALOGUING DATA ARE AVAILABLE

Library of Congress Control Number 2021052048

Front cover: (inset) The author with her son Brennan
in the hospital, 1997; background photograph © 2022 Shutterstock

Printed in the United States of America

Toplight is an imprint of McFarland & Company, Inc., Publishers

Box 611, Jefferson, North Carolina 28640
www.toplightbooks.com

For my son, Brennan,
who fought to win,
and in honor of my twin, Jerry,
the first and best

Finisterre

The road in the end taking the path the sun had taken,
into the western sea, and the moon rising behind you
as you stood where ground turned to ocean: no way
to your future now but the way your shadow could take,
walking before you across water, going where shadows go,
no way to make sense of a world that wouldn't let you pass
except to call an end to the way you had come,
to take out each frayed letter you had brought
and light their illumined corners; and to read
them as they drifted on the late western light;
to empty your bags; to sort this and to leave that;
to promise what you needed to promise all along,
and to abandon the shoes that brought you here
right at the water's edge, not because you had given up
but because now, you would find a different way to tread,
and because, through it all, part of you would still walk on,
no matter how, over the waves.

—David Whyte
In *Pilgrim* (2014), Many Rivers Press, Langley, Washington

Table of Contents

Preface

When my four-year-old son, Brennan, was diagnosed with leukemia, I was a cancer nurse, researcher, and educator. Although I mostly worked with adults who had cancer, I knew what to expect regarding treatment options, side effects, and how to navigate the healthcare system. But I had no training as a cancer *mom*. I felt responsible to advocate for my son and guide my family through treatment, yet I felt vulnerable like every other parent who fears losing their child. Fear of the unknown is a human condition. Uncertainty frightens and immobilizes us. Brennan drew pictures to process and share his emotions. I buried my feelings and flew into action.

My son survived his leukemia, but a decade off treatment, my fears came back to haunt me. The things we avoid have energy. I wrote this book to make sense of our experience and to finally face my fear of losing my son. Through my family's story, and my struggle to negotiate my roles as both mother and cancer expert, I share my personal and professional insights on survivorship, resilience, and healing. Brennan, too, shares his pictures, journals, and dreams. Reflecting on how illness shapes our lives and reframes our priorities is important to moving on with meaning and purpose. You, too, can learn to let go of the fears, guilt, and anxieties that haunt you in the middle of the night.

Because events in this book happened ten to twenty years ago, I relied on my journals, notes and photographs and my son's medical records to stir my memories and remind me of facts and feelings. Throughout his treatment, I wrote scenes and dialogue in my journal to help me capture and process my feelings, confusion, or uncertainty. As a researcher by nature and training, I did my best to validate experiences and confirm facts and put them in perspective as accurately and honestly as I could.

Although the treatment protocols today for children with cancer include many of the same medications, schedules and "road maps" have changed, and, in some cases, new medications have been added. Clinical trials continually evolve with the goal to increase survival and reduce long-term effects of both the disease and its treatment.

I have changed some names and identifying details to safeguard the privacy of those I could not locate or who chose not to be named. Others have opted to be included by name, and I thank them for sharing themselves with you. There are no composite characters or events, although memory has a way of blurring over time.

Introduction

Years later, long after treatment ended, I stood at the ocean shore as dusk descended with an unexpected swiftness. Blackness blanketed the bay, and I felt the same fear and isolation I'd experienced that first fretful night in the hospital. I peered into the darkness, expecting the horizon to orient me, searching for the line demarcating sky and water, insight and perspective, when suddenly the waves surged up over my knees, throwing me off balance. I grabbed for my husband's arm and backed up toward the shore. In my determined effort to find a beacon, I'd forgotten to pay attention to the moment.

PART I

The First Year
Getting Through

Fears are like shadows. They loom bigger in the dark.
—Thomas Moore, *Dark Nights of the Soul*

CHAPTER 1

January 9, 1997,
2:40 p.m.

Brennan lay stretched out high atop the pediatrician's oak examining table. Even at age four and a half he reached across the entire length. Half-reclining on his left side, facing me, perhaps watching me, he leaned on his left elbow and tossed every few seconds to reposition away the pain in his thin, long legs.

"Hi, Brennan, back again?" the nursing assistant said as she walked in, set down her tray of supplies, swiped his finger with the pungent alcohol swab, and pricked his middle finger with a tiny lancet. He watched, as if observing a science experiment, as the red drops defied gravity and rose up the capillary tube. He didn't cry.

After the assistant wrapped on a miniature Donald Duck Band-Aid, I asked if she could tell me what his lab results were from his last visit, two weeks earlier.

"I didn't bring him in," I said.

She nodded and went out to check for me. Moments later, she slipped in and quietly closed the door behind her. She hesitated and then recited, "His white count was 6.5, and his hemoglobin was 8.6."

"8.6?" I said, composed but incredulous. I knew that his white count was fine, but normal values for hemoglobin were at least 12 to 13 grams/deciliter. Anything lower meant anemia; a hemoglobin below 9 was serious. I looked straight into her eyes as the nurse in me tamped down the rising panic of a mother's worst fears. "Why weren't we told?"

She gave a sympathetic shrug and dashed out of the room.

I stared at the closed door. I wouldn't let myself consider the significance of the low value, so I focused on the lack of disclosure. Anger was easier to face than fear. Why hadn't they told Laurie, our nanny who'd brought him in just before Christmas? I'm certain she would have told me. Did they think it might be an error? I was afraid to believe that it could be real. I tried to breathe, to stay in the moment, ignoring the diseases shouting their textbook headlines. Just that morning I had considered infectious disease; I couldn't imagine a common virus causing sporadic fevers and intermittent pain. All I could do was wait for the new results. I stood next to Brennan, my hands gently resting on his legs. I took a deep breath and asked, "How are you doing?"

"Okay," he said with a blank expression.

I'd like to imagine that I was channeling energy from the universe to help his body heal or at least to disperse the pain in his legs and give him strength to tolerate it. I wanted my touch to reassure him, to tell him I was there for him. I wanted to be present for him, as I envisioned a concerned mother might be, thinking about how he must feel. Instead, my nurse mind churned with uncertainty, collecting and sorting the ambiguous facts and data, trying to tessellate the events of the past two months into some coherent picture.

CHAPTER 2

As the Seasons Change

The fall of 1996 had been a season of change, one where it seemed like the most important events happened when I wasn't paying attention. The structure of our lives shifted. Brennan started preschool; my husband Duane added evenings to his already full-time work schedule; our nanny of four years took six weeks off to donate a kidney to her brother; and in August we began a major house renovation.

Our compact, cedar shake Tudor was tucked back from the parkway in an established neighborhood of early twentieth-century homes, with large oaks and elms lining the boulevard. Across the street was a spring-fed pond surrounded by cattails and everything green. Wild foxes, deer and turkeys canvassed the backyard for seeds and nuts from the feeders. Yet we were only one mile from downtown Minneapolis where Duane had worked in banking since we'd moved from Chicago twelve years earlier. The Guthrie Theater, just down the street, had been our day trip cultural destination while dating in high school. We never imagined living so close to our past. And now we wanted more space for our growing family.

On the first day of excavation, four-year-old Brennan and his sixteen-month-old brother Tyler stood for hours in front of the living room bay window, hypnotized by the backhoe lifting and purging until three steep walls of damp, cool emptiness replaced the grass and rhododendron bushes of the front yard. When I came home from my teaching job at the university, Brennan immediately recited a play-by-play account of the day's progress. He leaned into the curved window jutting out over the hole and said, "Look how deep the hole is! They found these old bottles wayyyyyy at the bottom!"

He ran back to the kitchen, expecting me to follow, to point out three blue and green medicinal glass bottles drying on a towel on the kitchen counter.

Tyler stayed at the window, and when I came back into the living room, he pointed to the big yellow backhoe parked on the dirt ledge, facing the house. Its windows shone like eyes and its feet were extended out and locked into place, blocking the front of the hole. "You have one of those in the sandbox, don't you?" I said, and he nodded, both eyes fixed on the larger-than-life machine fifteen feet from his view. We didn't linger long, however, as an upholsterer and our nanny's mother were coming shortly. The boys didn't get dinner until after 8 that night. The evening routine was as disrupted as the front yard, the rhythm of life off-kilter.

Then, despite the backhoe's protective position, we awoke at 2 a.m. to desperate cries of "Help! Help!" The middle-aged newspaper delivery man had fallen into the ten-foot abyss.

My nurse antennae zeroed in on his pain and disability, while my responsible homeowner fury questioned every decision the contractors had made. I have always emphasized prevention and early intervention, in contrast to the crisis management choices of my husband, but somehow, in the flurry of events that season, I had fallen far short of my intent. Deserved or not, I felt responsible, and guilt seeped in through a riverbed of distraction.

There was little time for recrimination, however, as the following day our nanny went in for surgery and we flew off to Disney World with my parents on a planned escape from the construction chaos. I had two weeks off from work, and I was grateful for one last summer hurrah and to be able to retreat to a captivating "other world" with family.

Brennan loved the stimulation and excitement of all the Disney parks, but the waterparks were his all-time favorite, especially the water slides where he could whoosh down alone and plop with a big splash at the bottom.

"I want to go down the *big* slide!" he exclaimed as he pointed to the vertical drop slide that promised speeds of X mph.

"Not with me!" I preempted, not caring what the exact number was, as I eyed the bodies lying flat and whizzing down, arms crossed over their chests, water spraying out over the sides.

"Come on, Dad! Will you take me?"

"I'll take you," Duane said, "but you have to be tall enough, and it looks like you have to go down by yourself." And off they went to check it out while Tyler and I swam around like tadpoles in the shallow pool, with Grandma and Grandpa watching from lounge chairs in the shade.

In the Magic Kingdom, Brennan introduced himself to every Disney character he saw, danced with Tigger on the street, and posed for family pictures with Mickey. His favorite rides were steering the old Model Ts around the track and racing go-carts with Grandpa. "Let's go again!" he would shout as soon as they came to a stop. My father's clear blue eyes twinkled, just as they had when he and my mother had taken their four teenagers to Disney World in 1972.

The boys caught colds and coughed the entire trip, keeping us all awake at night. By the end of the week I was so exhausted my vision was blurred and my mind unfocused. Looking back, I remember less about our time in Florida than the crises that bookended it: first the newspaper carrier falling into the hole in our yard, and then, twenty-four hours after we returned, my father's massive heart attack.

I had barely unpacked when I found myself in the car with my three siblings, who flew in that night. We drove to the hospital four hours away in Wisconsin where my father had been resuscitated and taken by air ambulance. Regret pumped through my own heart. Just two days earlier, we had scoured the shops of Disney for my father's usual antacid, but I hadn't even asked him about his symptoms. He didn't go to the parks on the last day, and I thought he was just tired or needed time alone. *If I had only paid more attention, asked more questions, could I have saved the 50 percent of his heart that died?*

Four days later, after my father's condition had stabilized, I returned to Minneapolis on a Saturday at noon to find Duane sprawled across the couch next to Tyler's crib, the boys crawling over him, vying for king of the mountain. He looked at me with imploring, basset hound eyes, no doubt expecting rescue. Rather unsympathetically I asked, "Have you packed anything yet?" We had two days to move to an apartment before the construction crews broke through the front walls. His silence told me the answer.

The construction schedule reeled us forward into fall. We moved to the twenty-first floor of an apartment downtown, Brennan started his first preschool program at our church, Duane taught a business executive class four nights a week after networking all day, a new part-time caregiver filled in for our nanny, we made weekend trips to check on my parents, and I somehow managed to begin a new semester of teaching my graduate oncology nursing classes. All I could do was get us where we needed to be.

So when Brennan's preschool teacher called me with concern that he had impulsively swiped all the books off the shelf in front of the other kids, I suggested, "Maybe he's absorbing my stress." But then the leg pains started.

At Halloween, Brennan, dressed as a ghost, sat rocking on two legs of the kitchen chair, waving his arms as he talked to Grandma on the phone about the first bag of Halloween candy he was old enough to remember. "I got a *big* candy bar at one of the houses," he said. "Dad drove us up to the top of the hill, and there were lots of other kids." He didn't tell her about the leg pains that had been flickering on and off throughout his day, so maybe they weren't so bad. I stood in the doorway, snapped his picture and smiled, relieved by his energy.

The pain continued for weeks, intermittently and inconsistently, but he didn't complain. He simply rubbed his thighs and showed me, when asked, that the pain traveled from his hips to his knees. In both legs.

We moved back to our renovated home the night before Thanksgiving, with Duane transporting the kids and the cat while I taught my Wednesday evening class. The next morning, family arrived from out of town to join us for sledding in the snow and Thanksgiving dinner. I didn't have time to think about Brennan's symptoms, and I secretly hoped that life would go back to normal now that we were home.

In those first weeks after Thanksgiving, Brennan raced Tyler on Radio-Flyer scooters around an imaginary track through the new family room, calling out, "We're on the Indy raceway!" as they sped through the living room, kitchen, dining room and back around the loop. By Christmas, the dark purple velvet robe Brennan wore as the King carrying frankincense to baby Jesus in the preschool reenactment dwarfed his rail-thin body. Even his smile was crooked in the picture. I started to worry.

Brennan's leg pains were now interspersed with episodes of abdominal pain; neither could be explained by physical activity or bowel patterns. Fevers of 101 or 102° F would mysteriously appear and then disappear within twelve hours, without any symptoms of a virus or other infection. We made three visits to the pediatrician, but he didn't seem too concerned. It was easy for all of us to ignore symptoms that went away.

And then, on a trip to the Mall of America with his little cousins four days before Christmas, Brennan's fever spiked to 104°, the highest it had been. But again it was normal the next day. Laurie, our nanny, who had recovered from her surgery, offered to take him to the pediatrician, knowing how overwhelmed I was with having company and planning travel and holiday preparations. "Make sure you tell him we are going out of town for Christmas," I called out as I raced off to get grades in before the holiday break.

"He seems fine," the doctor told Laurie after drawing Brennan's blood and examining him. "Go have a good holiday."

It was the first and only time I let someone else take either of the boys to the doctor. I rarely even let Duane take them in alone. I always wanted to be there.

* * *

We were back in my childhood home in Wisconsin over the Christmas holiday, celebrating my father's continued presence in our lives. Rarely did all four siblings and families come home for the holidays. The fifteen of us posed for what we expected to be our last family photo with my father. As it happened, my father would live to see another thirteen Christmases. I didn't know that the person I really should have been worried about was my son.

The next day, Brennan stayed in bed in the darkened hotel room, his knees curled to his chest to assuage the abdominal pain. "I'll stay with Brennan," Duane offered. "You and Tyler go." I hesitantly agreed, thankful for the chance to be with my family and to escape in order to think more clearly about what to do about Brennan's recurring symptoms.

Tyler, bundled in boots, snow pants, and a bright gold jacket and hat, stood with me outside my family's nineteenth-century, white clapboard house, watching the big fluffy flakes of snow drape over the ceramic goose decked out in her red velvet cape, perched on the front porch. I was mesmerized by the beauty of the day, but all I could think about was Brennan's pain. I contemplated taking him back to Minneapolis because there was no pediatric care in this small town. But he had just been to the doctor a few days earlier. What would have changed? And only the emergency room would be open over the holiday weekend.

I resented the intrusion of the pain and worry invading the beauty of the day. Christmas was a magical season, meant to be celebrated with family carols around the piano and dinners and card games around the antique oak dining room table. I was an eternal optimist, always looking for the positive and expecting things to be okay.

Tyler and I, encompassed in a whirl of white, walked hand in hand down the middle of the dead-end street where I had played kickball and softball on warm summer days as a kid. We would wait, I decided, until after the weekend to go back to Minneapolis, unless Brennan got worse. Then we would leave immediately and go to the ER at home, which was only two hours away. It felt good to have a plan.

After spending all day huddled in bed wrestling the stomach pain, Brennan announced after dinner that evening, "I want to go ice skating!"

"Are you sure you want to go out, Brennan? It's almost eight o'clock, and it's only ten degrees above zero," I said, walking over to check the thermometer in the kitchen. He looked pale and weak, but was undeterred. He was anxious to try out his first pair of ice skates, a coveted Christmas gift.

We bundled up the five kids and drove to the local ice rink that seemed to shrink with each passing year. When I was in junior high, my best friend, and sometimes my twin brother and I, would skate for hours, swooshing in rhythm to the piped-in music, practicing leaps and twirls in the spotlight, pretending to be Olympians. Twenty-five years later the drama was gone. There was no music and no warming house with a pungent wood-burning stove. Snow pile shadows encir-cled the small rink, and a teaspoon moon silhouetted the handful of overdressed shapes skating forward in slow, awkward motion. No one came to Zamboni the ice.

At first Brennan let Duane and me support him, one on each side. Then he insisted on going it alone. He fell, got up, fell, got up, over and over. The rest of us skated around, pulling the younger cous-ins on a sled, secretly watching and saying very little. He wouldn't want us to call attention to his failed efforts. After about forty min-utes he threw up his arms and shouted, "I can't do this anymore!" He'd given it his best shot, but he had expected more from himself, and he rarely skated again. We didn't know then that he was anemic, that his hemoglobin was half of what it should have been, making his heart pump harder to get oxygen to his muscles and vital organs.

CHAPTER 3

Diagnosis

In the silence of the tiny exam room, I could finally see the child, my child, at the center of that frenzied fall season. I could now see how his pain and fevers had gradually increased in intensity and frequency, how he had fought the weakness, and how it now consumed him. My shoulders tensed. Why hadn't I been more concerned earlier? How could I let the distraction of the house renovation, our hectic schedules, and my work be more important than the health of my son?

Just that morning, his hand had shaken like an old man's when he handed me his Lego figure. His brow scrunched, his eyes averted from mine, and he silently and swiftly pulled it back and tucked it into the pocket of his navy blue sweatpants. Neither of us said a word. I don't know how I could have let that shared moment evaporate. I wish that I had swooped him up in my arms, held him close, and asked him how he was feeling. Instead, I gave him a quick, reassuring hug and set off for work.

It was Laurie, our nanny, who paged me out of a research meeting at noon and said, "I'm worried about your son."

I was worried too. "Make us an appointment," I said, relieved that she was taking action. I was never a diagnostician. I was a nurse who cared for patients with cancer after their diagnosis. And now I mostly mentored students and designed and carried out research studies. But I had carefully tracked and catalogued my son's symptoms, as any good scientist would. Not once did I consider cancer, my own clinical specialty.

I sighed, shifting my feet. "I'm sorry we have to wait so long, Brennan," I said as I lightly stroked his legs. "The doctor should be back soon. Then we can at least give you some medicine for the pain."

He quietly endured the wait, his eyes not meeting mine.

Although I didn't realize it yet, in that moment we were straddling two worlds: before and after. I would soon feel myself hovering in midair, simultaneously grieving the loss of a normal childhood for my son and working extra hard to keep life as ordinary as possible. But in that moment of waiting, I stood my place and clung to the moment.

The door latch clicked. The doctor abruptly walked in, sighed, and said, "He has leukemia." Just like that. No hesitancy, no pause. He was sure. The additional drop in hemoglobin to 6.5 that day was the pivotal puzzle piece.

"Which kind?" I asked, knowing that it mattered.

"A-L-L," he replied. Acute lymphoblastic leukemia, the more treatable type.

I nodded at the answer, pretending that my cancer knowledge might save my son. I didn't dare look at Brennan. How would I even begin to help him understand? I needed time to think, to sort out the implications for myself. And to retrace the signs I had missed.

The doctor lightly placed his hand on my back and asked, "Are you okay?"

I murmured "yes," convincing myself that I was. I had to be okay. My son needed me. I sat back down, feeling lightheaded, and took the piece of white prescription paper with the name of the oncologist scrawled across the top. The doctor had already talked to one of the two oncologists at the clinic. Later, when we got to the oncology clinic, I realized that he had written down the oncologist's first name wrong. He too must have been distracted. At a later visit he told me that Brennan was the fifth child he had diagnosed with cancer. Or maybe it was the fifth child with leukemia, the most common cancer in children.

I slipped the note in my purse, mentally retracing how to get to the hospital across town.

Brennan lay still, looking at us, quiet and observant. "Go home first," the doctor said. "Pack a bag."

"Just one question," I said, my eyes looking up to meet his. "Why weren't we told that his hemoglobin was 8.6 on his last visit?" I knew I sounded accusatory, but I deserved an explanation. The delay had given us Christmas together with my father, but a delay in diagnosis of leukemia could mean more aggressive treatment for my son or even his life. Now, even hours mattered.

He said something about the clinic not being certified to report hemoglobin levels.

Given the abnormal value, the conscientious procedure would have been to refer us to Children's Hospital to recheck the suspicious, but unverified, finding. It was too late to matter now.

The doctor turned to Brennan and said something like "I hope you feel better soon."

I let the triteness go. Silence would have been more uncomfortable.

I lifted my son off the table that was taller than he was, my hands almost circling his slender torso. With his feet firmly planted on the floor, he slipped his hand in mine as I opened the door into the dark, narrow hallway. I took a deep breath, and we exited our life as we knew it.

Chapter 4

The Plan

Laurie sat at the kitchen table and nodded her head. Yes, she could stay the night with Tyler. If I had been her, I would have rattled off a thousand questions, but her calm yet concerned demeanor helped me stay focused on my task.

I set out Tyler's evening meds for his asthma, but I wondered later, *Did I even say goodnight to Tyler?* He had been up much of the previous night with a croupy cough. At 2 a.m. I had held him in the hot shower to open his airways. He had never completed his whooping cough vaccinations because of neurologic reactions, and his risk for pertussis was always at the back of my mind. Here I was, more worried about his physical health than if he would miss me or his bedtime routine.

It was now after four in the afternoon and the clinic would close at five. I was outside, sandwiched between a low ceiling of colorless sky and crunchy old snow. I shuffled between the gray house and the gray car, tossing two haphazardly packed tote bags into the trunk while I used the other hand to dial number after number on the portable kitchen phone, trying to locate Duane. Where was he? He needed to know and he needed to be there. I was irritated that I had to track him down. The damp cold penetrated, but the fresh air helped me think. He was in between jobs, exploring new business opportunities, networking from a temporary downtown office without an assistant. He didn't have a personal cell phone. On a whim, I called the church and found him in a leadership meeting.

"Brennan has leukemia," I said. I paused. "Can you meet us at the pediatric oncology clinic?" Hearing only silence—or perhaps leaving no time for a response—I gave him directions to Children's Hospital, four miles away. The diagnosis had whipped away uncertainty, leaving me with a mission. I was an inexperienced parent but a competent cancer nurse.

Brennan climbed into his gray car seat in the passenger side of the backseat and buckled up. I mentally ticked off my list of overnight supplies as I buckled myself in.

As I backed out of the narrow, C-shaped driveway, one that always commanded my full attention, Brennan asked, "So, what's the plan?"

I tried to smile into the rearview mirror. I so wanted it to be just like any other day, watching him hop down the stairs in the morning, asking if we had any plans for the day. But his eyes were searching.

"We will go see another doctor, one who specializes in cancer," I said, well aware that I had used the word cancer instead of leukemia. He knew people who had cancer. He didn't know anyone with leukemia. I had no idea if he understood; it didn't occur to me to ask him or tell him his diagnosis. Maybe because I didn't yet believe it.

"We are going to the hospital. We will stay there with you until they come up with the best plan to treat you and make you better." I focused on one step at a time, the next one. It was all I could do, strapped three feet away from him, behind the wheel of a moving vehicle. If it were his brother in his place, he would have needed me to pull over and cradle him with love and reassurance. But what Brennan needed was an explanation, a plan. And what I needed was to get him the best treatment as quickly as possible.

A sense of urgency directed me, but a cloud of sorrow hung between us. I wonder if he too could feel the heavy weight of motionless air. He was uncharacteristically quiet. I expect that he sensed tension in my take-charge approach, my crisp words and staccato actions. I had no uncertainty about the plan. I had been trained to treat cancer. But my heart lurched in this new territory, seemingly stopping and starting at each red light, trying to comprehend what his little body would have to endure.

Part of me just wanted to get there, to start on the path that would take away his pain and cure his disease. Like Brennan, I needed a plan. The other part of me wanted to retreat back to before, to our old life.

*   *   *

We were at the oncology clinic within fifteen minutes, huddled together in another tiny exam room, the new doctor on my right and Duane on my left. Brennan sat cross-legged on the floor, outside the circle of informed decisions. The child life specialist distracted him with play while we conferred about his future.

After a series of questions, the oncologist asked, "Does Brennan have any siblings?"

The question sounded innocent. But it wasn't. The doctor was assessing the availability of a sibling bone marrow donor for a transplant. Fear and protectiveness for my round-faced, blond, curly-haired and blue-eyed Tyler shot through me. My mind silently raced: *He's not even two years old. How could I put him through that?* Then my fears turned to Brennan, the tall, thin, stoic, sandy-haired, blue-eyed boy seemingly intent on his play before me. Suddenly, I saw vivid flashes of the two sixteen-year-old boys with aplastic anemia whom I had nursed through bone marrow transplants in Chicago fifteen years earlier. I saw the tubes, the swollen tummies, the bald heads and puffy cheeks, and the sunken and angry eyes pleading for a release from the strict isolation rules. Both boys had died, each one comforted by familiar faces behind masks, touched through latex gloves. An image of my son on a respirator flashed across my view. I quickly gasped for breath and walked out of the memory.

"Yes, he has a brother," I forced myself to reply. "Twenty-one months old." And then I added, to assert his unavailability, "He was up all night with croup."

*   *   *

Where am I? Is this a dream? I asked myself every hour throughout that first night in the hospital as I tossed and turned on the stiff and crunchy vinyl couch placed next to Brennan's steel bed on wheels. I jolted awake every time someone walked into the room. I was ready to record any data, answer any question, observe any interaction, and process any problem. When the door closed again, I slipped back into restless sleep.

"Ow! Ow! Ow!" Brennan had screamed just a few hours earlier

as a calm and focused male nurse took three tries to get an IV into his little hand, clenched from fear and pain.

"I know it hurts," I said, stroking his head as I cradled him against my chest and his dad held his IV hand to keep it from moving. "It won't hurt after he gets it in."

After a day of seeking answers and direction, I was cornered by confusion. *Why did I allow his symptoms to drag on for so long?* I admonished myself during those dark, vulnerable hours of solitude and exhaustion. "Two months is the norm," the oncologist had said that day. But I wasn't the normative parent, was I? The past fall had been chaotic, far from normal, but I wasn't comforted by excuses. I had higher expectations for myself. Of course, now, after diagnosis, I could see how the symptoms pointed to cancer.

Cancer was my job, my career. Cancer was only supposed to happen to other people's kids.

I sat up to see Duane nestled into the recliner in the darkened corner, between Brennan and the window. We hadn't talked; one of us was always with Brennan. Besides, what would we have said? We were both introverted thinkers who needed time and space to process things on our own. After twenty years of marriage, we reverted to our comfortable roles of divvying up responsibilities, knowing what they were without having to announce them. For now, we were just doing what we were supposed to do. We were there together, comforting and loving and protecting our son in the only way we knew, by acknowledging our son's vulnerability and masking our own.

My thoughts tumbled throughout the night, one after another, testing me. I thought I should cry, but tears never came. I kept trying to make sense of the day's events and to grasp the significance of how leukemia would change our lives.

*   *   *

Within twenty-four hours, acute lymphoblastic leukemia (ALL) was confirmed by bone marrow biopsy, a procedure in which marrow is extracted through long, hollow, stainless-steel needles from deep within each hip bone. Another poke in Brennan's spine, a lumbar puncture, ruled out involvement in his brain and central nervous system, a common place for leukemia cells to hide. He had standard-risk ALL. Not "favorable," but not "unfavorable" or "high risk." Although his white blood cell count doubled every few hours that first night, it stayed under the 50,000-microliter cutoff that would statistically increase his risk and require more aggressive treatment. Waiting just one day might have changed his treatment plan and his prognosis. We had made it in time. I hoped that I could stop blaming myself for the delay.

We would find out a week or so later that the tips of his chromosomes 12 and 21 were translocated. Something had triggered a break and they had swapped places, resulting in fusion of their TEL and AML1 genes. There are numerous possible gene rearrangements causing leukemia, we learned, and this one was associated with a better prognosis. Approximately 25 percent of all children with newly diagnosed precursor B cell ALL carry this gene rearrangement.

Eventually, these children would get less aggressive treatment and still maintain a higher-than-average 90 percent cure rate—but this discovery was still emerging at the time of Brennan's diagnosis. We wouldn't benefit from it, and it wouldn't move the mountain that lay ahead.

*　*　*

We went face to face with reality the next day, our second day in the hospital. The treatment-deciding parent meeting was scheduled for 1 p.m. I raced back and forth between the hospital and home, intent on being present for Tyler, yet also trying to be at the hospital when the doctors made rounds or updated any plans. In between procedures and tests, Brennan and I played cards, drew pictures, watched movies and participated in interactive hospital programs. "Get here in time for the show, Mom," Brennan reminded me. "I want to see if I can win."

I had arranged for a guest lecturer for my classes and canceled meetings for the week so I could be with my family. On my way back to the hospital for the parent meeting that day, I walked outside into the cold January sun. It offered light but no warmth. I was startled to see my research assistant, who lived forty miles away, run up the sidewalk, breathless.

"Oh! I'm glad I caught you!" Lynne said before I had a chance to even greet her. She handed me a copy of a 124-page research protocol that outlined the steps of the clinical trial she was sure Brennan would be on.

As a researcher, I knew that clinical trials were studies that followed a defined protocol to compare the effects of specific treatments on survival and outcomes. The ongoing goal for cancer was to improve cure rates while reducing the side effects and late effects of treatment. I wasn't even sure Brennan would be treated in a trial. But because fewer children get cancer than adults, pediatric oncologists rely on national clinical trials to more efficiently collect data and test hypotheses. It's the fastest way to move the science forward.

"How did you know which one?" I asked, my eyes wide as I reached out to accept the document. Lynne had been at the hospital research meeting with me on Thursday when Laurie had paged me, but I didn't remember talking to her after that. How had she even known Brennan's diagnosis? Instant communication, with social networking, texts, and smartphones, didn't exist yet. Then again, I couldn't remember talking to anyone in the last two days. I didn't even remember calling and telling my parents and siblings, though I knew I had.

"It's the only protocol open for enrollment for pediatric ALL," Lynne said. "I couldn't go to bed until I found it for you." She had access to clinical trials that I had no clue how to retrieve; she knew I would feel more confident armed with information and a plan. I gave her a sisterly hug and slid into the car with Duane to head back to the hospital for the parent meeting.

I scanned the first few pages, but all I saw were clumps of letters organized in neat rows on a page. It was only a ten-minute drive to the hospital, but it was the first time Duane and I had been alone together since Brennan's diagnosis two days earlier. We must have talked about something.

Neither of us cried. We were experts at suppressing our emotions, and my tears always created an uncomfortable silence. When we talked, it was usually about our schedules, or the boys' schedules, or logistical plans for whatever house maintenance, event or vacation we were planning. We were both adept at doing, accomplishing tasks, checking off lists, and making things happen. We took turns reaching for our goals. For the first fifteen years of our marriage, one of us was always in school. I became pregnant with Brennan the month I defended my dissertation, and our focus turned to growing careers and raising children. Cancer was not in our plans.

Just as we walked into Brennan's room, the child life specialist rolled in a computer on a cart and challenged him, "Let's see who can capture the most Mario points!" Distracting Brennan was our cue to leave for the meeting. I turned and watched him excitedly scoot to the edge of his bed in front of the big screen. I hesitated. It was so hard to leave him. What if he needed me and I wasn't there for him? He didn't let on that he needed his dad or me. It could have been me who needed him more, or maybe I needed him to need me. Each moment with him was precious time together.

I forced myself to put one foot in front of the other. At least we were on the same floor, I rationalized, just down the hall. And he knew the plan. He would play and then we would be back.

Duane and I silently walked down the hall together, protocol in hand. We met with the oncologist and nurse in a small, square, white conference room with a round gray table and a white corded telephone on the wall. If there was a picture, I didn't see it.

The oncologist confirmed the diagnosis and genetic phenotype, the day's facts. The new FISH (fluorescence in situ hybridization) technology that would give us more detail on the DNA characteristics wasn't back yet. But that didn't determine treatment, just the survival odds.

"There is one clinical trial open through Children's Cancer Group for standard risk pre–B cell ALL," he said, confirming Lynne's findings. "There are four groups called 'arms,' one of which Brennan would be randomly assigned to." He went on to explain that the purpose of the trial, a large, multi-site research study, was to determine if a newer oral drug (thioguanine or 6-TG) would be more effective at increasing survival rates than the one currently used in the same pharmaceutical class (mecaptopurine, 6-MP). The study also tested if "triples" (three drugs injected into his spinal fluid at periodic times during treatment) were more effective than the single agent that was currently the standard of care in preventing central nervous system relapse.

He noticed the protocol in my hands and confirmed that it was the one Brennan would be enrolled in if we chose to participate. "You don't have to get treatment through a clinical trial," I heard him say. He was obligated to offer all the options. All I could think was *But it's because of the research that more than 80 percent of children with ALL now survive, when almost half of them died twenty years ago.*

Back then, in the early 1980s, I'd worked as a staff nurse at the Dana Farber Cancer Institute in Boston. The founder of the institute, Dr. Sidney Farber, had pioneered the use of chemotherapy to achieve the first-ever remissions of childhood ALL. Every day I walked past the first-floor pediatric clinic to take the elevator to one of the adult oncology units. I never lingered. The survival rates weren't much better on the adult unit, but at least most of the patients I cared for had lived longer than I had. It was because of Dr. Farber's drug discovery, and ongoing clinical trials like the one our oncologist had just told us about, that survival rates had inched their way up since then to hopeful percentages.

"The national trial opened eight months ago," Dr. Steve went on. "They will recruit over 2,000 children; it will take four to five years."

"How long will Brennan be on treatment?" I asked.

"Three years from the start of the first Interim Maintenance, which for Brennan should be sometime in early March."

I nodded, signaling him to go on. I wrote four pages of notes; seeing the plan scribbled out helped me grasp our new routine. The first twenty-eight days of "induction" consumed an entire page. The possible side effects of the thirteen intravenous, intra-spinal, and oral medications walked on to the next two pages. But in the lower right-hand corner, just before turning the page, I wrote: *Remission: < 5% blasts in bone marrow; 10^{13} leukemia cells down to 10^{5-6} in 28 days.* Ten trillion leukemia cells down to one million. I looked up and saw the oncologist's gentle brown eyes and steady, reassuring gaze. Remission was our mutual goal. We would know within twenty-eight days. The numbers would tell us.

At that moment, the immature, rapidly proliferating leukemia cells—the "blasts," which were untrained at fighting infection—were crowding out the red blood cells and platelets in Brennan's bone marrow. If we didn't treat the leukemia, he would die from infection, bleeding, or heart failure from anemia. The thirteen drugs used during the twenty-eight-day induction were expected to wipe out the majority of leukemic blast cells. The following three years of treatment would eradicate any stragglers—forever, we hoped. The earlier the remission, the better Brennan's long-term chance for survival. How could we choose otherwise?

"What if they aren't down to 5 percent by day twenty-eight?" I asked cautiously.

"Then a bone marrow transplant would be indicated."

I nodded and looked down at my hands. My shoulders sagged as the images of the two boys in transplant filtered back into my mind.

Duane had been quietly leaning back in his chair. I had been facing away from him, and I would have had to turn away from the oncologist to see what he was thinking, how he was responding. I turned when he asked, "It sounds like most of these symptoms are expected at some point. Do we continue with treatment as scheduled unless his liver enzymes go up or his blood counts go down too far?"

I was relieved that he understood. While I needed all of the details, he focused on the big picture, just like he did at work. A year later he would tell me that it helped him to know that I knew what to expect.

After two and a half hours, we both signed the informed consent to put our son on the clinical trial. It was a relief to have a plan, and yet it was a heavy anchor in our new world. We had just authorized the team to direct our family's destiny for the next three years and two months. By the time Brennan came off treatment, almost half his life would have been devoted to daily treatment for cancer. But an 80 percent chance for a cure was worth it. We would diligently follow the plan, the clinical trial "road map." I felt comforted by the years of research, the history of knowledge, and the commitment of professionals involved in this plan. I also felt captive to the new world we were navigating.

By the time we somberly walked side by side back down the long corridor to Brennan's room, steeped in our own thoughts, it felt as if an eternity had drifted by. The halls were quiet, though I knew that every room had patients. The staff bustled about, but I never felt rushed. I wondered how the oncologist and nurse had the entire afternoon to commit to a single family. I thought about the other families and wondered where they were in their treatment plans and how many had just had their lives transformed by a new diagnosis. *We can't be the only ones going through this*, I reflected, putting myself in my more comfortable professional role. I lifted my shoulders, ever so slightly, just for a moment. It seemed so much easier to be the nurse than the mother.

The next day we were told that the computer had randomized Brennan to the most aggressive arm of the protocol. They didn't quite say it that way, they simply said, "Arm B2." But I knew. He would get the newer oral drug, 6-thioguanine, and the three intrathecal meds, the "triples." The goal was to prevent central nervous system relapse and to inch up disease-free survival. On that day, if I could have chosen an arm, I would have chosen B2. I desperately wanted my son to live, and I believed that the more aggressive arm would improve his chances. The trade-off was that the side effects would be more acute and prevalent and the long-term consequences potentially more dire. I knew that, but at the time, survival felt more urgent.

"He will be in the hospital for six to seven days," the oncologist said. "We will start chemotherapy as soon as we can get a central line placed for infusions."

I understood the logistics. It was reassuring to be guided through the expectations one day at a time.

We'd faced one of the most important decisions of our lives, and yet the choice seemed clear. We gave our son his best chance for survival. We chose life, with all of its uncertainty and risk. The odds were in our favor. And then we moved forward, together, with the plan.

CHAPTER 5

The Training

Our son had an 80 percent chance of living through treatment. We had hope. And yet I was unprepared for the solitude of survival I carried with me.

Half a century earlier, my grandmother had lost hope. Her mental illness had manifested at age twenty-two, shortly after her fifteen-year-old brother, her closest surviving sibling, had died of diabetes on Christmas Day. There was no treatment for diabetes in the early 1900s, and the standard of care for mental illness and depression at the time was isolation, restraint, and institutionalization. It would be the 1950s before Thorazine became available. Although I never knew her, my grandmother and I were both women in our forties when we faced life-altering circumstances. The choice she made would influence my life.

She died at the hospital, hanging from the stockings she'd wrapped around her neck, her toes reaching down, inches from the floor, arms dangling in midair. I imagine her wearing a gray or brown dress, one with a collar—something typical of the 1940s and reflective of her depressed state. I envision her hands, wrinkled and worn thin by years of farm chores, kneading dough, washing clothes in buckets and wringing them on washboards, grinding grain, and foraging for wild mushrooms and blackberries, four children in tow.

She killed herself at a place she'd gone to in search of help. She was supposed to leave the hospital that day and go back to the private mental institution she had moved in and out of for three years. The repetitive cycle of depression without recovery had taken its toll. She was married, but her parents paid for her care. It was the best available treatment in rural Wisconsin at that time.

Her daughter, my mother, was twelve years old.

"No one ever told me how she died," Mom confided seven decades later, at the age of eighty-one. "They just told me that she died. I figured it out."

Mom was the youngest of four children. I can imagine that her family thought they were protecting her. And yet she was left on her own to make sense of why her mother had died in a hospital, a place intended to make one well. She must have felt very alone, and sad, and I would have understood if she was even mad. But she never shared her emotions. She buried them.

When I asked about my grandmother as a child, Mom would simply say, "She died when I was young." If I asked how or why, she would get quiet, her eyes dark and distant. Over time, I too forgot about the woman who would have been my grandma.

* * *

Seventy years after my grandmother's death, I took my mother to visit her eighty-nine-year-old sister in Montana. In my aunt's long, narrow living room, Mom and I sat, thighs touching, on the new love seat of the same rose, blue, and tan colors as my mother's couch back home. I looked around at the four stuffed chairs, the cane rocking chair, and the tattered walker next to the recliner, wondering how often my aunt had enough company to fill those seats. Her youngest daughter had driven 500 miles to see us.

Aunt Irene excitedly pulled out the historical issue of *The Holcombe Centennial: 1905–2005*. "I have to show you something. I marked the page," she said as she awkwardly reached over the arm of the walker to hand the black-and-white softcover book to my mother.

Mom paused, but she did as she was told and silently flipped open to the page marked with a lime green sticky note. There on the right-hand page was my mother's first and last name, printed in shaky cursive ink, and an arrow pointing to a girl in the back row, her shoulder-length hair clasped tightly away from her face. The class posed in front of a white clapboard schoolhouse. The photograph was simply titled "1942."

"Oh!" I exclaimed, jumping up to get a closer look. "This would be the one-room schoolhouse you talked about!" I was elated to recognize some small snippet of information I had stored over the years. Mom loved books, and whenever we would see an old country schoolhouse, she would mention having gone to school in one. The older kids had taught her how to read. But when had they moved to Holcombe?

"I think Mother is in the bottom picture, with the other parents," Irene said. "But I can't find her." She handed Mom a full-page-size magnifying glass and Mom found her in the front row, seated stiffly on a chair, her hair cropped short, a hat on her lap, arms tucked closely in at her sides. She faced forward, expressionless.

Irene then pointed to the "1943" photograph. Mom again posed in the back row, her face slimmer and framed with new wire-rim glasses, reminding me of myself at that age. Her mother would have died in January of that year.

"I think Dad is in there," Irene added, almost in a whisper. Mom quickly and quietly, although tight-lipped, pointed out their father. He stood in the back row, with only his face and hat visible. I was surprised that Mom could pick him out so quickly from the fifty tiny figures of parents and children attending the annual end-of-year picnic. I was secretly glad that he was present. It meant that he had been there for my mother.

"I could make copies for you," Irene prompted as she pushed herself up with both hands from her chair. "I might even be able to do it on my printer."

"I don't like to remember those times," Mom said as Irene bent over her to take the book. "It was hard for me." She looked up at her older sister as if she might not have gotten the message. My mother's lips quivered and her back tensed, but I couldn't tell if she was angry or just sad and regretful. She was unaccustomed to speaking her truth.

Irene quietly nodded and let the book settle on the table in the silence.

Later in the day, my aunt told stories as Mom quickly sifted through black-and-white pictures handed to her.

"Slow down!" I said, knowing I might never see them again. Mom mostly brushed aside my questions, seemingly frustrated at having to explain any facts, as if I should just "get it" and move on, just as she had.

Irene recalled two incidences of protecting her mother and her sister, my mother, from their father's wrath. "I didn't want him to hit my mother, so I stepped in between them," she said. Silence followed.

Back in the hotel room, Mom went straight to the bed. As she crawled in at three-thirty in the afternoon, her voice was strong and clear. "I don't know why Irene has to talk about that stuff from so long ago. She talks about all the bad stuff. I remember good things about my dad. Someone told me after my mother died that I would have to get up and make breakfast from now on. I remember waking up that first day after the funeral and starting breakfast. Dad came in and said, 'You don't have to do that, I can make breakfast.'"

She went on as I leaned against the wall at the foot of the bed.

"My dad was good to me, but it was our mother who we really relied on. I came home from school one day and she wasn't there— she was out on a walk or something—and I felt lost. I didn't know what to do. When she died, I had to rely on myself. Sometimes I seem selfish," she said, as if apologizing, "but it's just that I learned early on that I had to take care of myself."

"That's a lot to expect of a twelve-year-old," I said gently.

According to attachment theory, learned self-sufficiency is a natural response to rejection and loss. In the absence of consistent emotional support, self-protection and survival replace a sense of trust and security. With her mother in and out of hospitals for three years, and withdrawn and depressed even before that, Mom grew up with loss and abandonment. How would she know if her mother would be home, or emotionally available to her, that day or the next? She learned to rely on herself. She learned the task of "doing" at a critical stage of her personality development. It was her way of adapting.

After her mother died, instead of receiving comfort, my mother buried the memories and painful feelings she didn't know what to do with. What else would a twelve-year-old do?

Emotions may hide, but they don't disappear. They encode themselves in the brain's limbic system, where long-term memory, behavior, motivation, and a sense of smell also reside, which explains why responses and actions later in life can be driven by emotions long since buried.

We bury painful emotions to avoid feeling them. But, ultimately, it requires more energy to control the emotions than it does to just feel them. It took my mother seventy years, and her sister's coaxing, to peel back the outer onion skin of memory, and even then, she did her best to hold back. Her heart still closed to protect itself. She had silenced it for a lifetime.

Keeping stuff inside traps us emotionally. The heart is a vital energy center, and closing the heart blocks the flow of energy. When faced with uncomfortable feelings, instead of facing them and working through them, it's natural to overcompensate to avoid them, to control them, swinging the pendulum from one extreme to another. The pendulum is so busy keeping up the momentum of "doing" that it never rests at its center, where it can just "be," where the feelings can be acknowledged and felt and the fears released. It's not a coincidence that Mom developed stress cardiomyopathy, an enlargement of the heart resulting from stress hormones, at the age of seventy-two, while worrying about my father's own heart condition. Lack of attachment and nurturing at an early age influenced how she managed stress throughout her life. Closing her heart had become a habit, but like any habit, I knew it could be broken. I caught a glimmer of hope as I stood in the hotel room, acknowledging her anger, her fear, and her love. It took courage for her to share, and I tried to be accepting.

I was nineteen when she first told me how her mother died. We were sitting at the kitchen table talking about a health issue of mine. I didn't realize it then, but I think that she might have been worried about how I was handling stress. Years later, when Brennan repeatedly lashed out in anger in response to little things, she suggested, "Maybe he's depressed. I know he's only eight, but it can run in families."

It would be years before I could see how my grandmother's illness and choice influenced how my mother lived her life, how she parented, and how her patterns became mine.

*   *   *

When I was eight years old, I ran upstairs to my bedroom crying about some sibling infraction I no longer recall. After she finished cooking dinner, my mother came upstairs to my room, sat down uncertainly on the end of the bed, turned her head toward me, and asked, "Do you like to cry?"

What kind of question is that? I wondered then, although I tried hard to come up with an answer for her. She didn't ask me about my feelings or even about the situation that had triggered my distress. She asked about the visible evidence of the inner emotional turmoil. At that age tears flowed easily for me. No, I didn't like to cry; at least, I didn't like whatever made me cry.

A few years later, our four-year-old dog, Skipper, bit a little girl who had raced through our yard intent on a shortcut. She wasn't from the neighborhood; Skipper didn't know her.

As I walked home from school later that week, a neighbor boy, two years younger than me, ran up to me in the alley and said, "Skipper is dead. Your parents put him to sleep today."

I stared at him, my eyes welling up with tears. "No, they didn't," I replied. He seemed to be taunting me, bursting to share his secret news. I wasn't going to cry in front of him and reward his insensitivity. I was mad at him for his self-serving and flagrant desire to tell. But it was my parents who really merited my anger. They had used the same preemptive silence when they'd euthanized our first dog several years earlier. I came home from school to find Trixie gone. She had been old and sick. I remember feeling sad, but I was too young at the time to fully comprehend what I later perceived to be the unfairness of their approach. And now they had betrayed me again. I never got to say good-bye.

Even though I had three siblings, Skipper was very much my companion. I was the one who walked him most nights and who wrote poems about him after we'd gone galloping together through fresh-fallen snow. When the Catholic nuns at the neighborhood school complimented his shiny coat, I shyly thanked them, pretending I had some part in it.

I ran home feeling angry and confused. I spent the rest of the day and evening crouched in the dark, dank basement with the ancient octopus oil furnace, its big round arms extended out in every direction above me. As painful as the darkness was, I clung to the emptiness.

I avoided my parents for days afterward. Even an eleven-year-old can conceptualize death as final, and there was no excuse in my mind for not preparing me for my loss, if not involving me in the decision. They could have at least told me so I would have had a chance to say good-bye. I missed Skipper terribly, but even more hurtful was the lack of preparation and communication. They didn't offer comfort, and I had no intention of seeking solace from the people who had caused my suffering. I moved on alone.

No one talked about Skipper ever again. It was as if he'd never existed. My anger simmered over the years, like the fire generated deep within that furnace. When I admitted to my brother, four decades later, that it still hurt to think of Skipper and his untimely death, he told me that the girl Skipper had sunk his teeth into was the district attorney's daughter. I guess that was supposed to justify my parents' actions, but my heart wasn't listening.

I would come to realize that my mother left me alone to deal with my own grief after Skipper died because that was how she had handled her grief after her mother died. And it's possible that by distancing herself from her own emotions, she could not empathize with mine. I learned to stop the flow of my own tears. But the hurt remained even after the evidence dried up.

I didn't realize the implications of this subconscious decision to suppress until I experienced a soul retrieval session with a shaman forty years later. In the session, the shaman connected with three personas from my past: a three-year-old girl, collapsed from the exhaustion of carrying water from the well across the barren fields to fill the sadness she'd absorbed from her parents; a rebellious teenager, damming up the symbolic water in the mountain stream as the only way she knew to control the energy she constantly gave away; and a thirty-year-old white marble statue, frozen in time because the well water, the energy source feeding her soul, had run dry. Years of suppressing feelings and damming tears had blocked my own energy, the shaman said, manifesting over time as inadequate adrenal and immune responses. My adult self had run low on energy in part because of the beliefs I had clung to from an early age. I hadn't let go and I didn't know how to restructure my relationships. Just as my mother had, I had learned to rely on and trust myself, however unreliable or immature that self was in the moment.

I had learned early on how to survive. As the second, smaller twin baby, I was isolated alone in the hospital after birth. My twin brother had gone home with my parents and older sister while I fought alone to survive. And then we both fought for our place in a family with three children under the age of one.

Although my mother tried, she had little experience with emotions. And typical of the 1950s and '60s, my father, a stoic German, relied on her to handle anything regarding feelings. I didn't know to expect anything else. I learned to squelch my feelings and to survive on my own.

* * *

When I was sixteen years old, I worked at the front desk of our small-town hospital, admitting scheduled patients to hospital beds and triaging patients to the emergency room. There was something about nurses' intensely human spirit under crisis that pulled me into nursing and eventually to the field of psychoneuroimmunology, the science that explains how cells of the brain and body communicate with each other under stress and how emotions drive physical responses. I specifically wanted to know *how* a negative mood could suppress the cellular immune system's ability to control illness and cancer—and how positive emotional states might lead to healing or even longer survival. And I wanted to know how people found hope and meaning in illness and how they adapted to and rearranged their lives to accommodate adversity. I wanted to delve into the mystery of the human facing off between life and death.

My first patient to die had no family, or none that I was aware of. As a new twenty-four-year-old nurse, I walked into her room during the predawn hours toward the end of my night shift and saw a still and silent soul, alone and uncommunicative with the world her body still existed in. I felt a distinct absence, a nothingness that permeated the rectangular silhouette of walls and floor. The room was void of energy. My heart yanked. Her heart still beat. I had an hour before the day shift arrived and nothing urgent that needed to be done. I pulled up a chair and sat alongside her, gently enclosing her left hand with both of mine. She never moved. I sat, reflecting on the vibrancy of life and the stillness of approaching death. I wondered how it must feel to be alone at this time. Did she know I was there? Did my presence matter?

My patient took her last breath after I left work that morning. I never knew if she died alone. I only know that my heart was with her before she journeyed on. I was comforted knowing that I had taken the time to care and reassured that I had allowed myself to feel. Through her I had glimpsed the value of being fully present, of experiencing "being with" rather than "doing for."

Over the years, a subtle force guided me to uncover and reframe the denial and silence I had carried with me through childhood. Still, despite all my efforts to counterbalance my early training, this history of buried emotions, unexpressed grief, and learned self-sufficiency, patterned from generations before me and planted into my limbic system, accompanied me into the hospital when Brennan was diagnosed. Logically, I understood. Emotionally, under stress, I regressed.

CHAPTER 6

The First Week

Chemotherapy induction started on the third day of hospitalization. Outside, it was nine degrees below zero, with a brisk and biting wind that zapped through my core. Inside, the fluorescent lights and cheery phlebotomist illuminated the first step of the designated "road map," the treatment schedule that the clinical trial had plotted out for us on paper.

Everyone tossed around the term "road map" as if we knew what it was. To the staff it was as commonplace a phrase as "vital signs," but I wasn't familiar with it. A road map wasn't needed in adult oncology, where, at that time, standard treatment plans typically involved two to three chemotherapy agents given on the same day every two to three weeks. The recurring schedule wasn't hard to track. Pediatric clinical trials like Brennan's, however, called for specificity, with doses adjusted to body surface area (calculated by weight and height), and with eleven or more medications staggered daily, every other day, three times a week, weekly, or every three to four weeks. Once our children went home after six or seven "induction" days in the hospital, we would be responsible for the schedule.

Each landscape-formatted page mapped out twenty-eight-, fifty-six-, and, eventually, eighty-four-day courses of treatment in tiny, eight-point font, four columns of short blank lines synchronized to medications across the page. Each chemotherapy agent had a corresponding line for the date due and the actual date given. (Treatments are sometimes delayed because blood counts are too low.) The two right columns spelled out the labs, procedures, and assessments that were to be done before administering the drugs and any comments or reactions observed. The bottom third of the page explained a list of asterisks and the fine print of how to administer the drugs, the specific dosages by age, and when to withhold treatment. It was overwhelming.

I think most parents, like me, focused on the first two columns: the list of what meds to give on what day and when to bring their child back to the clinic. I admit that I never read the entire parent manual handed to us in a three-ring binder, but I did scour each road map. Once home, I placed it on the refrigerator to check and double-check each drug and dose. I carried a copy with me, and I consulted it before scheduling work meetings or other appointments. The road map, upon which our son's name was embossed in capital letters in the upper right-hand corner of every page, literally mapped out our routines.

One of the oral drugs had specific directions to avoid giving with milk or dairy products. The asterisk at the bottom of the page read, "Give at least one hour after PM meal, without milk products."

"Does that mean no milk products at dinner too or just at bedtime, when he takes the 6-TG?" I asked Sara, Brennan's nurse. Brennan craved cheese and ice cream and shunned soy and rice substitutes, which had casein, a milk protein, in them anyway. How strict should we be? I wonder if I was more compulsive than most parents. There was little clarity on the directions. We later discovered that some parents were told to avoid milk and others weren't even aware that milk reduced the drug's bioavailability by about 30 percent. It turns out that many children metabolize this class of drug with wide variability, so perhaps other factors were more important, like taking it at night rather than in the morning. It was hard for Brennan, but we held our ground through meltdowns and avoided dairy every night. I wanted to get it right.

So it was that we started on the first page of the twenty-eight-day road map on that frigid January day, the path that would define our lives for the next three years and two months. The blank lines on the page seemed to blink like a cursor waiting for action, urging us to just *get started.*

"You will feel better once we start treatment," Dr. Steve reassured Brennan as he watched my son rub his long, thin fingers up and down his bony thighs. "It's the leukemia cells that cause the pain."

Cancer cells multiply exponentially each day. One thousand cancer cells replicate to one billion cancer cells in a matter of hours. We needed to kill them, soon. But chemotherapy is not selective. It kills the normal, healthy, growing cells at the same time. Cells that replicate faster die faster—like the lining of the gut, hair follicles, and white blood cells. The consequence is nausea and vomiting, hair loss, anemia, fatigue, and infections. The trick with chemotherapy is to destroy a larger percentage of cancer cells without completely wiping out the normal cells. Treatment for leukemia and lymphoma is even more delicate because the blood and immune systems are critical for survival. Wiping them out completely ensures death.

The urgency I felt to start treatment was tempered by the uncertainty of what to expect. Or the certainty. I knew exactly what patients typically experienced with each of the thirteen drugs Brennan was scheduled to receive. But I also knew that every individual responds differently, and although we were informed of the entire range of possible consequences, from hair loss to loss of life, we wouldn't know how Brennan would tolerate the chemotherapy until he received it. We had to be prepared for everything. Or at least I felt I needed to be.

We had made our decision when we signed the consent form. Now we had to put our trust in the oncology team to guide us forward, step by step. I coached myself to stay present in the moment, to take one step at a time, just as I had advised my adult cancer patients over the years to do. It wasn't hard; I was overwhelmed thinking beyond any given day. So we did what 2,000 other families facing leukemia that year would eventually do: we began to march down that road map, jumping from line to line and column to column, until all of the black lines were filled in with completed treatment dates. January 11 was the first "actual" date, ready or not.

* * *

Brennan's first intrathecal chemotherapy took place on Monday morning, day four. Duane and I sat on the floor with him in the pre-op area, playing a bead maze, waiting for that first intrathecal injection to be delivered between the vertebrae in his spine, directly into the fluid that cushioned and protected his spinal cord and brain.

As the team of four anesthesia staff walked into the room, I got up quickly. Too quickly.

"Whoa, I'm feeling a little lightheaded," I said.

A female intern stepped out and brought me back the standard four-ounce sealed container of orange juice and two little packets of white sugar. She silently handed them to me. Her response seemed automatic, and I wondered how many other moms she had rescued with sugar. I gave her a questioning look, but we exchanged no words.

A few deep breaths might have also done the trick, but I drank the orange juice and pocketed the sugar, and soon I was standing inside the sterile surgical suite, trying hard to ignore the whirs of the equipment and to focus on my son through my cognitive haze.

The anesthetist and oncologist shepherded us along.

"The milky liquid going into his intravenous line is Propofol," one said. "It's quick and short acting. Brennan, you will fall asleep, and when you wake up, your parents will come in to see you."

The thick, milky anesthetic (the same one that killed Michael Jackson thirteen years later) slowly swirled into Brennan's intravenous line through the port-a-cath that had been surgically placed into his upper right chest. The medication would mix with his own blood, then proceed directly into his heart. It was safer this way and less traumatic than starting an IV line in his arm each time.

Duane sat on the shiny steel gurney and held our son, his strong, secure arms completely wrapped around Brennan's lean frame. Brennan bravely braced for the uncertain, saying nothing, and then he slowly slunk back into his dad's embrace. Moments later, his body went limp.

Everyone moved quickly and efficiently. I kissed Brennan, stroked his cheek, and whispered in his ear that I loved him, reassuring myself. Duane and I hesitated at the door, looking back. I watched as my son's chest rose once, his eyes closed, oxygen mask dwarfing his face. I saw a part of us lying still and defenseless. I wondered if he felt as powerless and vulnerable as I did. Did he know that we were on his side? I breathed in, turned away, and let the automatic door close.

The surgical waiting room buzzed with activity. "Who is the

patient you are waiting for?" the voice of the stout and "all-business" volunteer echoed. "Have a seat. We'll call you when they call us."

I was restless. I had lugged along reading for my class preparation. It sat in the bag. The television cheers were deafening as Bob Barker called out for the next contestant on *The Price Is Right*. It was noise where there should have been silence. I wanted emptiness, for my surroundings to mimic how I felt. I was certain that I didn't belong there. I was being ordered around. Wasn't I supposed to be part of the flurry?

I sat in a chair facing the glass door, where the light darted in and I could watch for the doctors. Duane sat next to me and then quickly got up, saying he was going to make phone calls in the hallway. I nodded. Doing nothing was especially hard for him. He was a business executive who was used to moving from meeting to meeting, making prompt and confident decisions and taking action. Waiting for things to happen was not in his repertoire. Him sitting next to me and tapping his foot or fumbling with his pen or papers would just aggravate us both.

The chair next to me sat empty. A murmur of surprise escaped me when Nancy, my friend and former lab tech, walked in and positioned her thin, fit, older self in the chair next to me. Suddenly, everything else vanished. Nancy didn't say anything. She didn't have to. Her daughter, Betsy, had died of ALL two decades earlier, when only half of kids diagnosed with it survived.

Nancy was a consistent presence throughout Brennan's treatment. She would leave work in the middle of the day to walk across the street to bring us her church youth group pizza for dinner and to play putt-putt golf with Brennan in clinic. She would tap the golf ball into the crocodile's open mouth with the same intensity and precision that she used to run precious blood samples through the flow cytometer, measuring the number and type of lymphocytes in patients with cancer. She was there when I most needed to laugh and when Brennan needed someone other than Mom to entertain and distract.

Nancy's presence was reassuring, and I didn't have to pretend around her. I later wondered what she gained from these visits and if spending time with us reactivated the memories of her own daughter's treatment. What were her regrets?

*   *   *

After about an hour, after Nancy had gone back to work and Duane had reappeared, Dr. Steve walked in the door to reassure us that all had gone well and that Brennan was in recovery. When he led us into the post-op area, I felt out of place, even intrusive, in the way. I tried not to look at the rows of steel beds lined up with kids lying flat in every one. I was being Mom in that moment. I kissed Brennan and reassured him that we were there. I don't remember anything else from that day. But I do remember his resistance to subsequent bone marrow biopsies and spinal taps.

Brennan quickly caught on that having his dad carry him to the elevator meant another procedure that would separate him from his parents and make him feel dizzy or nauseated upon waking from the anesthesia. It was like he put on his armor and raised his shield, ready for the fight. "I'm not going for the back medicine!" he would yell as Duane carried him and I corralled his flailing arms and legs and pushed the elevator button, carrying the requisite buddy and blankie tucked under my arm. It took all of our physical strength to get his forty pounds of resistance to the pre-op area for the weekly, and then monthly, and then every-three-month crusades. Some days I wished someone had a buddy and blanket waiting for me.

For years Brennan talked about how the intrathecal injections were the hardest thing he had to go through. When he was eight years old, just two months after coming off treatment, he admitted to an audience of cancer professionals, "The hardest thing about having cancer was getting the back medicine. I knew I would wake up not feeling good. And I really hated it when they put the Propofol in my port. It made me very, very, very dizzy, like a tornado swirling around." And when he was thirteen years old, he wrote in his English assignment, "I hated bone marrows and I tried to get out of them so many times. I would always sob and sob because it was so bad. It seemed like I had to have one every day, because once I would get over the last one, I would have to have another one."

I don't remember sobs; I remember determined resistance.

*   *   *

Brennan was our first-born child, the one who determinedly came into this world at the exact stroke of the big hand on the twelve. It was as if he had emerged precise, focused, and ready for action. When he was just four hours old, in the soft light of night, I awoke to find him watching me from his bassinet. His large, quiescent eyes observed me lying on my side, facing him at eye level, hands tucked under my head and denting the goose down pillow encased in vibrant red, pink, and blue impressionist flowers.

His eyes didn't question, they didn't ask, they didn't show. My newborn tranquilly watched me watching him. In one of those rare moments in an entire lifetime, he had caught me sleeping and I had caught him dreamily just observing. The silent serenity warped time.

Four years later, he was the one dwarfed in the hospital bed, with his red and black Mickey Mouse pillow tucked under his pale, sunken cheeks and vacant blue eyes, his faded blankie with sailboats and his mouse buddy dependably by his side.

The transformation from one hospital visit to the next created a chasm so deep I feared looking back. My heart ached for what was and had been, and yet my mind seemed determined to replay visions of his pride as he kicked his first soccer ball, hit baseballs from the front yard, swung his dad's golf club, and leapt solo from the low dive. And then, at age four and a half, I watched his energy dissolve into each unfamiliar and invasive procedure. Over and over I glimpsed the joy of his brief childhood, his infectious laugh and dancing eyes, drift further and further away, until I could never fully retrieve them. Instead of joy, memories brought heartache.

* * *

Each day in the United States, forty-three parents are told, "Your child has cancer." Nine of those children will have leukemia. As a parent, and even as an oncology nurse, I never ever imagined that my child would be one of the 0.004 percent. We weren't alone, but I sure felt alone.

At no time in my few years of parenting had I ever considered that my child might die. Optimistic by nature, I had always expected the best of everything. There was no vulnerability, no hesitation, no risk communicated between us in those wee hours after his birth.

And over the years, we never compromised on safety. We wore seat belts and bike helmets, cooked organic food, avoided cancer-causing nitrates, breathed and drank filtered air and water, and, as much as possible, shunned environmental chemicals. Not because I feared cancer down the road, but because I lived daily with the effects of chemical and food sensitivities. I could not have knowingly prevented leukemia, and now I could not predict or control what the future held for my son. I lived with a new awareness, a new vulnerability, knowing that I couldn't protect him from the hurt of having to go through cancer treatment.

*　*　*

Over his course of treatment, Brennan turned to art to help him make sense of his new world. His media were diverse—markers, crayons, chalk, watercolor, and oils. Bold color was the single pervasive element.

He drew a house his first day in the hospital. Thick, black, tar-like strokes completely sealed the two-story structure. Six bold, red, jagged spears jutted out from the side and the steep roof, apparently aimed at anyone or anything that got too close. In between the spears, a proportionally large blue figure clung to the outside of the roof, reaching in toward a smiling yellow shape inside the peak. There was no one else inside.

"It's a birdhouse," he told me. "There is a little yellow bird inside. There is a warning to stay away."

He signed the picture in the upper right-hand corner and drew an arrow from his name directly to the peak. It was if he was making sure I knew that he was the little yellow bird.

Two days later, he drew another birdhouse. The red pointed spears still surrounded the frame, now bordered in light strokes of lime green. The little yellow bird still smiled and roosted inside the peak of the roof. Each extremity of the figure had a solid round dot on it, perhaps signifying all the "pokes" it had had.

Brennan pointed to the thick, black arrow, which again was aimed toward the roof but was a bit off center this time. He whispered to me, "The window is the only way in." I envisioned him choosing whom to let in and whom to deny access to, an attempt to exert some control over his new world.

He had printed "Mom" and "Toy" under his name. I pointed to the stack of presents piled up outside of the house, perhaps reflecting his effort to bring back the Christmas fun he had just missed out on. "There are toys and lights—to look pretty for Mom," he told me as he looked at the colorful page.

My four-year-old was thinking of me, his mother, at a time when he could so easily be consumed by his own survival. Since his birth, Brennan's eyes had revealed an old soul, but I had never felt his empathy until now. When he was an infant, my family referred to him as "baby Jerry." He resembled my twin brother in features,

but even more so in temperament. He was fiercely independent and always seemed one step ahead of us, his parents. He knew what he wanted, but he had to learn how to communicate that to us. So he challenged himself from day one, just as my intellectually gifted brother always has.

"Thank you" was all I could manage as I hugged him from behind.

Years later, when he reflected back on that first week in the hospital, Brennan wrote, "I liked to draw

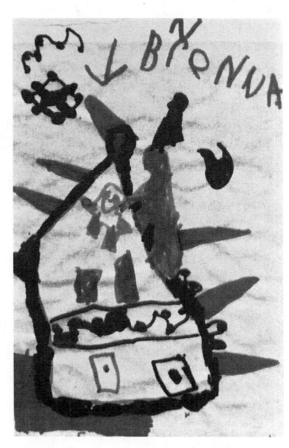

Brennan's house, day 1, diagnosis.

because it was the only way I could think of to let my true feelings out. To this day, my mom still uses my pictures for her talks, and even though I'm a perfectionist, I still look at those pictures and like them. This is probably the biggest thing I did in the hospital because I learned a way to express myself."

His drawings opened the window to his feelings, helping me to understand, to see his new life from his view. I wanted to pay attention, but I didn't know how to ask. My four-year-old showed me the way.

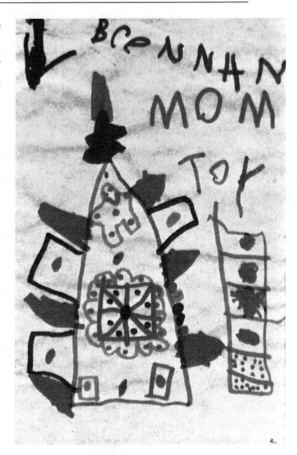

Brennan's house, day 3.

*   *   *

On good days, Brennan tried to fool everyone about his age. It wasn't hard. He was off the charts in height and verbal skills. Like an entrepreneur, he capitalized on the opportunity.

"I'll bet you can't guess how old I am," he teased every staff member who walked into his room.

A long pause would typically be followed by "Hmm, you look seven years old to me. I'm usually pretty good at guessing ages. Am I right?"

"Nooo," he would say with a grin, "I'm six and a half!"

And then came the standard reply: "Are you really? I was so close!"

"You're wrong!" he would say, laughing. "I'm four and a half." And he grew two inches and two years just then. I wondered if he were trying to convince himself that a six-and-a-half-year-old could handle life-and-death drama more stoically than a four-and-a-half-year-old.

*   *   *

The week in the hospital was well orchestrated and routine for the hosts, but a basket of uncertainty for us. "There's a new family with standard risk B cell ALL in room 722," I imagine the nursing staff reporting between shifts. "Mom's an oncology nurse," they no doubt added. I was unaware if my background influenced the care they gave my son or the way they interacted with me. I felt as uncertain then as I imagine other parents must feel. And I expect that the staff empowered all parents to take responsibility, whether we wanted to or not.

"Hi, Brennan, it's time for your medicine," the twenty-something nurse chirped as she walked into the brightly-lit room with a syringe half-full of liquid prednisone, standard formula for a four-year-old who could not yet swallow pills.

"I'm not taking it!" Brennan shot back.

"How about if we put it in some applesauce?"

"No! I don't like applesauce!"

"Then let's try pudding!"

"I hate pudding!" he replied, while I nodded affirmatively.

"Well, then, I'll go get some chocolate. How does that sound?"

I wondered how many more options there were and if this was expected defiance for kids learning a new mandated routine in a setting that offered few choices outside of flavors. She came back into the room with the syringe full of thick, syrupy chocolate. That would be some mouthful of goo. Which is what Brennan apparently thought too as he hesitantly but cooperatively let her squirt a tasteful into his mouth. He immediately dispensed it right back out over the bedside table and onto the bed linens. From then on, he would insist he never liked chocolate.

"Well, let's let Mom try!" was her still cheery but a bit more subdued reply as she walked out of the room to get a new dose of prednisone without chocolate. She came back, handed it to me, and left, apparently trusting me to follow through. Maybe she thought I would feel more comfortable without her watching. I honestly didn't know how to get my son to take the bitter-tasting prednisone any more than she did. My adult patients were much more compliant, I mused. Had she left me with this responsibility because I was a nurse? I wanted *them* to take care of him while we were in the hospital. My time was coming soon enough. At that moment, I really just wanted to be a mom.

"What should I put it in?" I asked Brennan.

"It doesn't matter, I won't take it!" he replied.

If he hadn't been so weak and ill, he might have fought longer, but eventually I wore him down and he swallowed the prednisone right from the syringe, chasing the bitter medicine with teaspoons of sweet and silky vanilla ice cream. That worked for the remainder of the hospital stay.

A few weeks later, on another sub-zero day, I resorted to straddling his captured body on the cold hardwood floor in the kitchen, trying to squirt the syringe full of prednisone down his throat, hoping that he wouldn't choke and that I wouldn't be the recipient of an erupting volcano. Afterward, abhorrence of my strategy overwhelmed the relief I felt at my relative success. I relented. I calculated the odds; they must have tested these trials with other kids who resisted. How far from the norm could he really be? Maybe if he actually took them all, his dose would be too much, I rationalized.

Shortly after, our nanny Laurie taught him to swallow pills. *Smart*, I thought. Laurie had him practice with pea-size balls of bread, Duane coached him with empowering imagery, and I measured out doses. Within a couple of months, by the age of five, Brennan was a master at swallowing pills—when he chose to. (I quickly learned to unfold and inspect the wadded-up napkin in the garbage can.) By the time he completed treatment, he boasted to an audience of 2,000 cancer practitioners, "Now I can take up to ten vitamins or pills at a time! My mantra for taking prednisone was 'I'm *big*, I'm *tough*, I'm a *grizzly bear*!'" He had come a long way since that first day in the hospital.

Our four-year-old had suited up in armor to face his fears. He tried on roles as if they were costumes. He grew from a tiny yellow bird, hiding inside, to a tall and wise warrior and sometimes a grizzly bear. In the midst of trying to grasp my own loss, uncertainty, and fears, I tried to understand and honor his.

Everything swirled inside me that first week. My professional understanding see-sawed with emotional intensity. I couldn't find the center, the lever, to balance my familiar roles with my unspoken fears. I'm not even sure I knew what I was struggling against. I was focused on just getting through. Duane probably was, too. He is a man of many thoughts, but few words. He might have been as afraid of the unknown as I was. I would never know because he didn't share feelings, and me sharing mine made him uncomfortable. So I shoved it aside for later, and later never came. We inhabited our own emotional orbits and just kept marching along. It was a time of getting through. The road map directed our actions but advised very little. I knew how to lead the army into battle, but I had no idea what to do with the effects, my responses and feelings.

CHAPTER 7

Finding Our Way

During that first week, when I was still navigating our new routine, I stopped in at our neighborhood coffee shop on my way to the hospital. After all, it was what I had always done on my way to work before Brennan's diagnosis. I had driven by every day now for three days; I was always in a hurry, consumed by my hesitancy to leave Tyler and my urgency to see Brennan and catch the doctors during morning rounds. On this day, however, a parking spot opened right in front of the café, and I swerved in. I salivated for that powerful punch of strong, black espresso. It was my first detour into public view.

I rushed through the door and then abruptly stopped. I had run into an invisible glass wall. Time stopped, and then fast-forwarded. I watched outlines bustle about serving coffee, tea, and signature scones and cinnamon rolls, a normal routine of their day. I had watched it one thousand times. But on this one thousand and first time, I asked myself, "What is normal? And what am I doing here?" I watched as the predictable world went on around me. I stood just inside the door, dazed, unsure of how I fit into this new world—or, rather, the old world, the one that had changed overnight.

I realized then that I could never go back. It was like how my golf swing changed after golf school. The swing that drove the ball straight and narrow, right down the middle of the fairway, disappeared. No matter how hard I tried to recapture the old swing, I realized after an entire season passed that I just had to move forward with the new one. I sometimes still wish I had the old swing back. The ball may go farther now, but it's unpredictable, harder to control, and it lands out of bounds more often. The old swing, like my former life, was reliable and safe.

"Can I help you?" the barista asked.

"Me? Um, yes," I said, not realizing that I had queued into line. I had been watching him, wondering if he would notice the sadness in my averted eyes, my sloped posture. At other times I might have disguised my grief, offering a fleeting, flashy smile. But the weight on this day was too heavy to hide. A part of me wanted him to ask how I was. I really wanted to unwrap and peel off a layer, to unburden some of the weight. But my eyes couldn't meet his. My mind swirled with different scenarios of what to say, how to say it. "Thank you," I said and carried my Americano in a small white paper cup, like a candle, back to the hospital.

The next time I went to get coffee, I simply rode the elevator down six floors of Children's Hospital. I watched as a group of five female staff, dressed up spiffy and chatting amiably, stepped in. I slunk back in the corner, making myself small. On a normal day, I might have listened, smiled, or even nodded in agreement. But on that day, during the first week of my son's diagnosis, I didn't want to know about their lives or their jobs or what their conversations meant. It was unsettling standing outside and looking in.

I wondered if I would ever feel like one of them again, like the nurse who cared about patients' lives. I could only think then of the uncertainty of Brennan's future and our life as a family.

I didn't know what the next day or the next week would bring. I had no idea when I would go back to work. The future daunted me. I couldn't see ahead, and I couldn't go back. I wanted to be the nurse who cared, and yet I was the mom caught in the corner. How could I be both? How silly of me to think I knew what cancer was about. Oh, I knew that I would see things differently, more clearly, over time. My patients had taught me that. But in that moment, the uncertainty felt foreign, murky. How was I to live with all the questions when I was used to having the answers?

* * *

Tyler, too, had to make sense of the change in his life. His big brother, a domineering and steady presence, was suddenly not there.

There was no one to ride the scooters or to entertain him at lunch. Tyler's response was to stop eating and playing.

He clung to me in the morning. "I need to take a shower, Tyler," I repeated over and over as he gripped tighter. So I took him into the shower with me, his little naked body tensely clutching mine, shutting his eyes against the rain pouring down.

On the third day Laurie strategically asked, "What have you told Tyler?"

My mind raced through scenarios of the past few days. My breath seized. As a quiet toddler, he didn't have the words or the inclination to ask, and I hadn't thought to tell. I immediately scooped him up and sat on the couch with him.

"Brennan has leukemia. He is sick and in the hospital," I told him. "The doctors and nurses are taking good care of him and he is getting medicine to make him feel better. He will be coming home, soon, we hope." I felt his sigh as he nestled into me. I measured my breath to keep from sobbing.

After several minutes I grudgingly said, "I am so sorry, Tyler, but I have to go back now to the hospital to see Brennan. I will be home tonight."

I felt as if I straddled two continents, my long legs stretched over the expanse of ocean. When I left for the day, Tyler was sitting on the bare family room window seat, staring out over the cloak of wintry white, as if waiting for color to come back to his world.

*　*　*

By the end of the week, Tyler's croupy cough had finally subsided; he was now allowed on the oncology unit. We walked slowly through the halls, allowing him time to absorb the sight of children his age being wheeled down the hall in wagons, intravenous poles trailing behind, driven by a parent. We took in the foreign smell of alcohol and antiseptic and the surround sound of voices, call bells, and ringing phones. I tried to imagine what a twenty-one-month-old might see. He had always been an observer of life, noticing much of what I might miss. We walked hand in hand to Brennan's room. I pushed open the heavy wooden door with the glass window, too high for Tyler to see through. His eyes zeroed in on the rumpled bed, occupied by Brennan's blanket and buddies, but no Brennan. He stopped and hesitated, his eyes scanning the inanimate balloons, cards, and pictures that filled the room. Suddenly, he heard Brennan's spirited and distinctive voice reverberate from the bathtub. Tyler giggled with glee, and like a butterfly in flight, he flew into the bathroom.

* * *

As a child, I was afraid of the dark. I imagined ghosts hiding and watching me. I saw images reflected in the ancient dresser mirror, shapes slipping around corners or through doors. Darkness hid the fears I could not see. I would sleepwalk at night and turn on the lights.

"Mom!" I would call out. "I need a drink of water!" What I really needed was a reassuring human presence.

As I grew older, I tried to understand why the dark seemed so ominous. I logically concluded that if I couldn't see it, I couldn't prove that it existed. And why, then, should I be afraid of something that didn't exist? If something was there, then I should confront it, get to know it, not hide from it. Not knowing only dramatized my fears.

One summer evening in the late 1960s, a childhood friend and I were startled to see lights in the sky as we walked home from playing tennis in the park. We walked faster, then slower, and eventually ran the last few blocks into my house. "There are lights outside following us!" I exclaimed to my two brothers, who met us in the kitchen.

Intrigued, they went outside to investigate. Both of my brothers were problem solvers, destined computer geeks, masters of code. After about ten minutes, while my friend and I waited, talking of aliens and spaceships and George Orwell's *1984*, my brothers sauntered back in with smirks on their faces. "It's a spotlight," they said in unison. They even determined that a vintage car festival had brought this new innovation to our hometown of 11,000 residents.

Identifying the unknown allayed my fears. When it wasn't possible, I acknowledged them. "You don't have to slither about. I'm not afraid of you," I whispered to the shadows, the ghosts, and sometimes even people on the street at night, who turned out not to be as scary as I imagined. I learned to comfortably share their space.

Of all the dark nights I had ever experienced, none were like those that swallowed me that first week in the hospital. I couldn't pretend that nothing was there. Cancer had shown its face. It was my fears that hid. And I didn't go looking for them; I wasn't sure what to do if I found them.

Some years later, when it was safe, I picked up Thomas Moore's book *Dark Nights of the Soul*. He describes how honoring these dark moments can be healing and can lead to new understanding of life's meaning. The purpose isn't to move quickly through these dark places, he says, but to have a view of life that includes the darkness. As our eyes adjust to the dimness, we begin to see more.

As Moore describes it, the light shining through the darkness, the light of healing, comes not from our ego but from our solar plexus. The ego tries hard to dictate events; the solar plexus seeks to understand and to feel. The only release from the pressure of the dark night is to let the process take place, to remain in the present, not bound or deluded by the past nor imprisoned by the future. "Fears are like shadows," he writes. "They loom bigger in the dark."

A comfort zone didn't exist in the dark. I wished that I could flick a switch and shine a light on the things that moved around us at warp speed, but that would just reflect, like bright headlights in fog. So I tried to take each moment as it arrived, in all its haziness.

It wasn't easy to just "be" rather than feel I had to "do" or even "see." At night, as I lay awake in bed, I tried to call on my past training in imagery and hypnosis, breathing in rays of white light—omnipresent energy from the universe—to cleanse each cell of my body and reignite the candle in my solar plexus. Some days the light flickered, and other days I couldn't even find it.

I lingered in the darkness for the first two weeks, where just surviving had its purpose. The universe moved on and I didn't. It wasn't like some gravitational force holding me back. It was me who resisted hopping back into the centrifugal momentum of life. I might have felt some refuge in the world I inhabited, but I think it was more inertia. I floated in space, my mind struggling to understand and to make sense of our new reality.

Just that year, I had finished a research study on hope. During a series of interviews over eighteen months, thirty-two patients with cancer had told my research team that having hope gave them the energy to face each day and to move forward with life, despite the uncertainty of how long they would live or how many symptoms they would endure. They relied on their inner strength, determination, and positive attitude, as well as family, friends, and healthcare professionals. They said that they needed "to know that I am not in this alone."

Hope also meant finding meaning and a purpose to living in the moment while simultaneously anticipating survival, whatever the odds. This emphasis on survival had surprised me, until Brennan was diagnosed.

Just a few weeks after his diagnosis, I went to visit my friend and colleague, Karen, who was home in hospice care, dying from advanced breast cancer.

"What are the odds?" she asked outright.

"Eighty percent of children survive," I said. "I try not to think about the 20 percent who don't."

She nodded as she sat up a bit in her chair, draped in a white blanket, her Irish Setter lying attentively at her feet. "I believed all along that I was in the 10 percent who would survive metastatic breast cancer," she said. "It kept me going, believing, having a purpose."

Karen had relapsed within two years of her first diagnosis, which seemed fast for breast cancer. She continued teaching while undergoing more chemotherapy and radiation for bone pain. Some of the 80 percent of childhood ALL survivors would also relapse and face treatment all over again. I couldn't imagine doing this twice when I was so far from getting through it once.

Karen died six weeks later.

Darkness is a part of life, as it is a part of every rotation of the earth. But some nights felt blacker than others. I couldn't just step outside and get perspective when I was mired in the muck. Karen and the patients in our study didn't ignore the despair or seek an unrealistic escape from the present. Hope wasn't wishful thinking. It was work. Their own self-determination and fortitude, along with support and caring from others, gave them hope and a reason to live.

They trusted the process to unfold. Light follows dark; hope emerges from despair. Somehow it just does.

*   *   *

Brennan came home after six days in the hospital. The pain in his legs had resolved, and he had more energy and enthusiasm after a blood transfusion and beginning chemotherapy. Tyler had certainty, routine, and his playmate back in his world. Duane got to sleep in a real bed again. I focused on getting through each day.

On our first day home, I videotaped the boys riding their Radio Flyer scooters around the new loop through the family room, barging through the bouquet of balloons that had followed us home from the hospital. They raced, laughing uproariously, as remnants of ribbon snagged the wheels and trailed behind like memories. Although I smiled and laughed along, I cry when I watch the video clip now, thankful for that bittersweet moment in time.

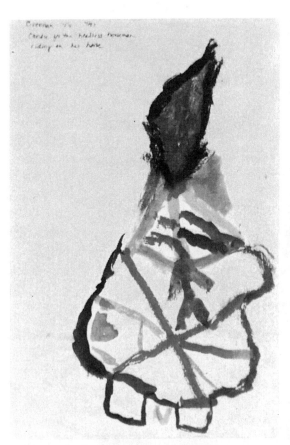

Brennan's headless horseman.

*   *   *

Not long after, Brennan showed me his abstract drawing of a triangle shape with two legs. The colorful figure, framed in brown, had an arrow for a heart and a bold, blue diamond, encased in strong, black lines, perched on top of its point.

"What is this picture of, Brennan?" I asked.

"It's the headless horseman," he said, as if I obviously would recognize the figure from reading the tale to him night after night. I had never liked the dark story, but it enthralled him.

"I gave him a candle for a head, to help him find his way," he said.

CHAPTER 8

New Identities,
New Perspectives

"My son has leukemia," I found myself telling the cashier in the checkout lane at Target, as if to explain the eight boxes of mac and cheese and nine pairs of three different sizes of boys' elastic waist boxer shorts I had stacked onto the moving belt. Brennan had gained five pounds the first month of induction, almost 15 percent of his body weight. He craved high-fat, salty foods. Most of the weight went straight to his tummy, thanks to prednisone's uncanny ability to store fat in the abdomen.

Explaining the unusual purchase seemed logical to me. And yet I could have been any mother buying boxer shorts and lunch for *three* hungry boys. What did the cashier care? I appreciated that she, and subsequent unsuspecting cashiers, just nodded their heads and allowed me to test out my new identity.

After two weeks away from work, I knew it was time to return. I struggled with the decision. It wasn't so much *if*, but more a matter of *when*. I didn't really perceive an option, as there was no one else to teach the oncology program. And I carried our family's health insurance, which had preexisting condition clauses. Sure, I was aware of the Family Medical Leave Act, which would allow me twelve weeks of unpaid time to be at home with my son. But that would leave my students dangling in the middle of their programs.

A few acquaintances (not my coworkers) suggested that I take the time off, but that didn't empower me. It felt more like them telling me what they would do. I was fortunate to have built-in flexibility with my job. No one said anything about the hours I worked or didn't work or the meetings I missed.

I called my twin brother Jerry, who was a university professor at Western Kentucky.

"I only go into work three days a week," he said. "Those days are crammed with classes, office hours, and meetings, but it gives me the other days to stay home and work on my research and writing. Could you just go in to teach and meet students and skip the meetings?"

I laughed. We both knew how antagonistic faculty meetings could be, and they rarely moved the agenda forward fast enough for us. We wanted our discussions to be meaningful, philosophical, or at least purposeful, leading somewhere enlightening, not mundane. Jerry was a conceptual economist who tested and applied mathematical and statistical formulas. I had chosen to study and statistically analyze the complex interactions of the body and mind. I never realized how similar we were until we both became teachers. Our students were always our priority.

During our first faculty meeting of the semester, I again questioned my decision to go back to work. We were discussing curriculum changes, a topic that always sparked controversy. I sat next to a colleague toward the front and center of the large classroom, watching the charged words volley back and forth over my head as faculty bobbed up and down like wound-up jack-in-the boxes. The clock's hands ticked into the second hour as I stared down at my folded, idle hands. The questions were reasonable, the tone ingratiating. *What am I doing here?* I wondered. *What purpose does all this bickering serve? My son fights for his life and my colleagues fight over dollars or the right to be right.* Even though I realized what was most important in my life, I didn't change anything, other than taking my brother's advice and skipping faculty meetings whenever possible.

Before we had children, work gave my life meaning. I loved the puzzle of science, the passion of nursing, the intrigue of cancer. I was at the forefront of my field of research. I wasn't ready to give it all up after training for thirteen years to get that far.

I had joined the faculty when Brennan was three months old. I was now a mother of a child with cancer who faced three years of treatment and a faculty member whose tenure would be up for decision during that time. I had two road maps, Brennan's and mine. Work provided some immunity from my new reality. I could never escape cancer, but I still could be the expert.

My graduate class was heading into week four of a ten-week course, "Psychosocial Issues in Cancer." Ironically, my first class back was "Family Adaptation to Cancer." The day before class, I entered my 100 square feet of office—crammed with two desks, four shelves of books spanning two corners, two file cabinets packed with course assignments and research documents, and a pile of "to read" manuscripts and journals teetering in a thigh-high stack on the floor in the corner behind the door. I ignored it all and sat in the small rectangle of empty space in the center of the room, rereading the journal articles I had assigned the students. The teacher in me jotted down bullet points, information that I deemed especially relevant from my new perspective, while the parent in me wondered, *How are we doing? Have I thought of everything? Are we normal?*

I grabbed a pencil and checked off responses to the questionnaires I had copied to hand out to the class. I had used these coping assessments in my research. They provided an objective and quantitative measure of how well a person or family with cancer was coping. After the initial crisis, most people tend to use a combination of the following: (1) cognitively reappraise the situation (find meaning, focus on the positive, feel grateful); (2) do something specific to resolve the distress (advocate for self, seek information, plan and organize); and (3) regulate emotions (use humor, cry, hide feelings, seek support). Some strategies are deemed more helpful than others.

I tried to avoid the term "coping." It felt so black and white, so judgmental, like you either cope or you don't—you either pass or you fail. Maybe it's just the harsh, hard consonant sounds. Or the feeling of being judged. I don't think I detested the word as much before cancer invaded our lives. I'm on the other side now.

Some strategies, like denial, avoidance, and emotional distancing, often get a bad rap, labeled as ineffective or even potentially harmful. I initially agreed with the experts, until one of our studies showed that women with breast cancer who tended to be "feelers" and who responded to stressful situations emotionally rather than cognitively or behaviorally "coped" better (according to the assessments) if they distanced themselves from their feelings of loss and grief. Stepping back and separating from the emotional intensity helped these women focus on the difficult decisions surrounding their treatment. I can imagine that setting their feelings on the shelf was hard for them, given how they naturally responded to situations.

I wondered what the "thinkers," like me, Duane, and even Brennan, would be better off doing. Too much analysis could get one stuck. I was too close to the situation, however, to have perspective.

As I read through the instruments, I ticked off "agree" to many items. *Sure, I worry about my other child; fatigue is a problem because of the cancer; I do live day to day because I cannot plan for the future; I am living on a roller coaster; and of course no one understands the burden I carry, unless they have been there.* I went on to the next instrument. *Yes, I am trying to maintain family stability, keep things normal, show that I am strong, take care of the medical necessities at home, and work at outside employment. And of course I believe things will work out. They always do, don't they?*

I couldn't sit still and I was talking out loud to myself. "Of course cancer has a major impact on families. Who would expect otherwise? So why does it feel as if we are expected to be positive-coping-super-role-models? Is it only me who leans toward answering 'I agree'? After all, I *want* to be doing well. Is it my German-American mindset to act strong and resilient, or is it my upbringing that taught me to sweep negative feelings under the rug of my consciousness? Where in this empowering do-it-yourself healthcare system are the resources to help us parents feel balanced and sane and capable while we do it all? And where, oh where, is the opportunity to just chuck it all and break down?"

I missed it, I suppose. Perhaps I was too busy trying to do it right.

I don't remember my total score on the questionnaires, but I recall taking them very seriously. I wanted to make sure that I had considered everything, but I also expect that I overinflated a few answers, just to make sure I was doing okay. If a patient or caregiver recorded a low score, I might look for signs of anxiety, depression, withdrawal. I would recommend a therapist or chaplain to help process feelings and find other, perhaps healthier ways to gain perspective, to cope. There was little information on how spouses and families adapt, only statistics on the higher-than-average divorce rate. I couldn't go there. I had to focus on the moment, on today.

There I was, looking for a number to tell me how I was doing. Why couldn't I trust myself, my own feelings? If the uncertainty of my new identity or my new role made me insecure, what would it take to feel more confident? Did I need someone or some assessment to tell me how I was doing?

Brennan, too, had to adapt to his new identity at a time when he was just learning who he was and how he fit into his world. Instead of playing basketball or baseball or building snowmen outside, he stayed in and played cribbage or board games and drew. For the first month he was too busy, too tired, and too sick to go to school or have play dates. He was the same child—I tried hard to see that—but he had a new dimension to his identity. At a time when most kids are eagerly tackling new tasks, sharing activities with friends, and trying things without the help of adults, he was spending his days at home with his family or at the hospital with a new set of caregivers who poked and prodded him and gave him medicines that made him sick.

Germs became our monsters in the dark. This was Brennan's only year of pre–K, though, and we wanted him to experience peer relationships and a structured school environment before starting kindergarten in the fall. I seriously considered holding him back a year, but he was tall for his age and he tested ahead of his peers. I wanted him to fit in.

The child life specialist and his nurse set up his "staged" return. Sitting in a chair in the front of Brennan's class, a puppet-size doll on her lap, Vicki explained what leukemia was, how Brennan got his treatment through a central line, and why he was bald. Brennan sat between Sara and Vicki and proudly lifted up his shirt to show his classmates his port-a-cath, which bulged under the still-red scar just under his right clavicle. Sara explained that leukemia was cancer and that you can't "catch" cancer like you can colds and flu viruses. But because Brennan was at higher risk for getting sick from these viruses, Sara showed them how to sneeze into their bent arms at the elbow, rather than their hands, and wash their hands with soap while singing "Happy Birthday" to themselves. (The teachers later reported that they celebrated lots of birthdays that first week back.)

The class listened to Vicki, entranced. Then they peppered Brennan with questions and commentary: "What does it feel like when they poke you?"; "How long were you in the hospital?"; "My neighbor had to go to the hospital"; "My grandma has cancer."

We didn't make a big deal out of resuming routines. I went back to work, Duane went into his office most days, Laurie and Tyler went to music class and adhered to their routines, and Brennan returned to school. He was four, and his job was to explore limits with courage and confidence, test out his identity with friends and peers, and engage in and direct play. He would learn self-control and gain confidence. At least, that's what the child development theorists said.

I'm sure there were times when he had doubts and lacked self-confidence, as all kids do. I think he overcompensated at times, trying so hard to fit in. Or perhaps it was the steroids, ramping him up like the Energizer Bunny, making him impulsive and reactive.

"It must be so hard for Brennan," one of his teachers admitted at his spring conference. "Sometimes he acts impulsively. Last week he got so frustrated he knocked down the bridges they were building, right in front of the other children." She paused. "We don't know whether to set limits, as we usually would, or to allow more flexibility with behavior that is most certainly a result of what he is going through."

"I know how that feels," I said, empathizing with them and yet secretly glad that I wasn't the only one witnessing his outbursts.

"He isn't as accepted by the other children now," she went on. "Some of his classmates seem to avoid him, and he is left out of some small groups at play time. It doesn't really seem to bother him, though. He goes off to play by himself."

Part of me felt reassured. He was adapting. But the other part of me ached for him, wondering how he felt about being left out. Was it a good thing that he retreated? Was he withdrawing to avoid interacting, further isolating himself from his peers, or was this his way of emotionally distancing himself to protect his vulnerable psyche? I wrote in my journal after the conference that I wanted to talk to him, but I wasn't sure how to bring it up. I didn't want to suggest that he might feel like an outsider or feel different from his peers. But who was I kidding? What would I be protecting him from?

Cancer was a part of his life, of who he was. By the time he started kindergarten six months later, he had learned to control his impulsive responses at school, even while on prednisone. I can only imagine the effort it took to maintain his composure all day.

One of the pediatric nurses in class one night commented on how much more mature and insightful children with cancer are. "They become great philosophers," she said. Which made me feel better, because Brennan already was a grand thinker. I tried to see this experience as a learning process in his early life. It would shape who he was, although I had no idea at the time how he would adapt. Hearing that there was a positive effect, any positive outcome to this life-altering and grueling experience, encouraged me. *Perhaps,* I thought, *it is through these difficult situations that children discover their strength and their courage.*

*   *   *

A few weeks after going back to school, Brennan drew a picture of "My Family." On a big sheet of golden yellow paper, he colored the four of us in crayon, off-center to the left. I was on the far left edge, outlined in red with a green face and hair. Brennan stood next to me, in between me and his dad. He, too, was outlined in red, with red facial features. The tall stack of hair he added on himself made him just taller than his dad. The real-life Brennan was bald by then, and he was half the height of his father. Duane was outlined all in black, with black eyes, nose, and the customary bowl-shaped smile. Brennan was the only one with arms, twig-like snowman arms, stretching out to touch my cheek on one side, reaching for his dad on the other.

"Where's Tyler?" I asked.

"He's right there," Brennan said, pointing to a tiny yellow figure—barely visible on the yellow page, just taller than the belly buttons of the three of us, and with no outline and no discernable facial features. I couldn't tell if he was smiling like the rest of us. With a red pen, to match Brennan's script, I printed "Tyler" next to his figure. I didn't even ask for permission. I just wanted him to be more present. He was almost two years of age, and Tyler's task was to learn to trust

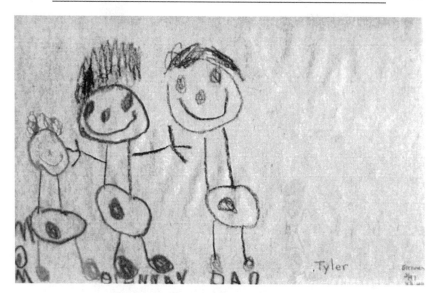

Brennan's drawing of his family, preschool.

his world, to know that his family was predictable, reliable, and consistent. I was offended by his seemingly inconsequential role in Brennan's worldview, even though it was a normal childhood perspective.

I tried to understand and to remember where Brennan was coming from, how he felt when he drew this picture. He made himself bigger than life, boosting his self-confidence at a vulnerable time. And he was the one reaching out to his parents. It was as if he was connecting us together on his behalf.

Brennan would tell me later, as an adult, that living with cancer was just what a four-year-old learned to do. "I didn't know any different," he said. "It was just part of my life."

* * *

Day twenty-eight of induction arrived. *Remission: 0.4% blasts,* I wrote in my journal. Less than 1 percent of Brennan's bone marrow was now inhabited by immature leukemia cells. In just twenty-eight days, those thirteen drugs had wiped out almost the entire population of 94 percent blasts. They had done their job.

As momentous as the day was, wiping out the cancer cells was only the beginning. We had to keep them at bay; we had to kill every single one so that they could never replicate again. And that required more treatment over an extended time, killing generations of newly minted blast cells. Still, I breathed a huge sigh of relief; we were on the right path, the drugs were working, and we had avoided a transplant, for now. And now was what mattered.

CHAPTER 9

Why Cancer?
Why Now? Why Us?

"How are things going?" Brennan's nurse, Sara, asked as she sat next to me in the clinic room after his first "consolidation" treatment appointment. Vicki had whisked Brennan away to play something fun. It was just Sara and me, alone.

Sara sat at my side, leaning forward as I talked. I felt an intense need to process the past before I could move on to the future.

"I've been thinking more about why Brennan got leukemia," I said.

"What are you thinking?" Sara asked quietly, her thin, delicate hands folded together on her lap, just in front of her barely visible baby bump.

I launched into a discordant litany of events, things that could possibly explain a genetic translocation, a leukemia trigger. I had contemplated them all over the past week, surprised by their existence as they flitted in and out of my awareness. Now they spewed out with volcanic intensity.

"I don't know, there are so many things, like my exposure to pesticides, chemotherapy, radioactive isotopes, electromagnetic waves, or the mycoplasma infection I had the year before I became pregnant. Did any of these play a role in his leukemia?"

"I don't know. Tell me more," she said calmly.

Sara wasn't leading me on; I was under no illusion that she had the answers. By listening, she allowed me to sort out and weigh the evidence that snaked its way in and out of my consciousness. I wish I could have ignored it. Why did I always have to spend so much energy trying to figure things out? Even Sara's presence blurred in my frenzy to focus on the evidence, to dive into the outlandish idea that I may have had some role in my son developing leukemia.

Since finding out that Brennan's leukemia cells carried a 12;21 translocation, I had been thinking about what could have triggered these chromosomes to swap tips and then replicate unimpeded in his cells. Had I passed along aberrant genes or a predisposition toward mutations? Or had I exposed him to something in our environment, either while pregnant or after his birth? Evidence suggests that genetic errors acquired from environmental exposures occur during pregnancy. Translocations can also occur as random errors in DNA replication. It could have just been chance. But is it a random event that 25 percent of children with ALL have this particular (TEL-AML1) translocation? Once the possibility struck, I fixated on knowing.

One month later, Dr. Mel Greaves, professor of cell biology and a director at the Institute of Cancer Research in London, would give a talk at my university on the molecular genetics and etiology of pediatric leukemia. In their genetic testing of identical twins, his team found that children who get ALL as infants are unique in that they have just one gene rearrangement on chromosome 11. Leukemia in older children, in contrast, is genetically diverse, with more than 200 detected DNA alterations. For these children, like Brennan, a "two-hit theory" explains how an irreversible gene mutation first occurs during pregnancy (initiating event) and is followed by an exposure or a condition that spurs the genetically altered cells to replicate (promoting event). Getting cancer requires both the initiating event (first hit) and the promoting event (second hit). It also requires the right timing and the right dose, making cumulative exposures over time more potent. The two-hit theory explains why some children may have genetic alterations but not get cancer and why the peak age of leukemia occurs a few years into childhood rather than at birth. The mutated cell sits dormant until the second triggering event, or the right accumulation of exposures, activates it and causes illness.

According to this theory, either a random error or an environmental exposure triggered the 12;21 translocation of Brennan's B cells during my pregnancy. And then, closer to his fourth year of age, something turned on or activated the expression of these genes, allowing the genetically altered B cells to reproduce, uncontrolled, until they consumed 94 percent of his bone marrow, four times the expected amount.

The "second hit" could be a common infection that triggers an immune response. Like hungry tiger cubs bracing to pounce on their prey, the primed B cells may recognize and attack the pathogen, but they aren't mature enough to kill it.

Just two months before the onset of his leg pains, Brennan caught a nasty virus that triggered a lingering cough and chest congestion. Tyler caught it, too, and both boys were sick throughout our late August trip to Disney World with my parents.

Most children develop adequate immune responses when exposed to common illnesses in the first few years of life. Their immune cells practice. Mature B cells even remember some pathogens so that they can pounce faster with the next exposure. Children who do not develop normal immunity and who are more likely to get leukemia tend to be firstborn children who have less exposure to other children and hence less exposure to viruses. They are often healthy until diagnosis, presenting with a history of fewer than expected illnesses in the first year of life.

When Brennan was an infant, I told his pediatrician that I thought my breast feeding protected him from illness. He nodded but said, "He's healthy because he isn't exposed to other children." These predisposing factors remain predictive, and there is continued speculation that viruses trigger the promotion of leukemia in children who have the genetic predisposition.

If gene mutations alone were not enough to cause cancer, then some other random error, environmental exposure, virus, or faulty immune response had contributed to Brennan's onset of leukemia. Instead of narrowing down my ascribed culprits, as I had hoped, my investigation convicted them all. Even if my exposures weren't triggers, they could be promoters.

* * *

Pesticides came first. Duane and I moved into university housing on the East Coast on a sultry August day of 94 degrees and light rain.

The elevators stopped on every other floor, skipping ours. It was the last apartment available, and we hadn't anticipated the fierce competition to secure university housing months before school started.

The cockroaches moved in after us. We lived directly above the convenience store, and interior walls made for easy access for the critters. We refused to let the staff spray our apartment because we were harboring a cat in a no-pet building. And because I worked night shifts, I shooed away the maintenance men whenever they pounded on the door or walked right in, waking me during the day.

At first we ignored the pests. But when the cat began to refuse to sleep on the floor and I repeatedly woke up to spiny legs scurrying up my exposed arm, we tramped off to the local Star Market and picked up the most vicious-sounding do-it-yourself roach bomb we could find.

The foggers killed the roaches just fine—until a new batch hatched or migrated up from the store.

I found out later that we had exploded Dursban (chlorpyrifos) into every crack, crevice, and misaligned cupboard and drawer in that 350-square-foot space. Organophosphate pesticides were later banned from household use in the United States and Europe, although they would continue to be sprayed on fields of fruits and vegetables and nests of mosquito larvae in parks and public places. Chlorpyrifos is a neurotoxin that irreversibly inactivates acetylcholinesterase, an enzyme essential to nerve conduction, and its acute effects are often lethal (think sarin, a terrorist weapon). The effects of low-level, chronic organophosphate exposures are not completely understood (i.e., not studied), although immune disorders, autoimmune diseases, and lymphoma cancers are linked to these pesticides in animals and humans. They are blamed for a 50 percent rise in lymphomas in farmers between 1978 and 1992, the same period of time we used them. Several other studies during the 1980s found a three-fold incidence of leukemia in children whose parents worked with or were exposed to pesticides in the home. More recent animal studies link organophosphates with lower T-cell immunity and chromosomal breaks in DNA. Someone is finally paying attention.

The cat and I developed food allergies simultaneously, shortly after we moved out of the apartment and back to the Midwest. It wasn't until Brennan's diagnosis, though, that I linked the cat's allergies to mine and both possibly to the Dursban.

Duane didn't develop food allergies; he isn't the allergic type. I inherited an impressionable immune system, growing up with asthma and airborne allergies. I would find out later that I also had a cytochrome P450 defect that prevented my body from breaking down the chlorinated toxins. Eventually, my confused immune system would be both deficient in B-cell antibodies and overreactive toward its own cells, resulting in frequent infections and extreme fatigue, lack of thyroid and adrenal hormones, and autoimmune disease.

Brennan's quantitative immune system eventually looked normal, but he would always have an inability to fight off infections or mount an adequate immune response to vaccinations. I don't know if his leukemia is pesticide-related. I do know that it happened as the result of an uncontrolled over-proliferation of immature, non-functional B cells. We both struggle to fight off infections. Brennan's disease was life-threatening; mine is merely life-altering. But the coexistence is likely not coincidence.

* * *

I also considered the irony that I, an oncology nurse, would have a son with cancer. And then I remembered my daily handling and administering of chemotherapy drugs, exposures that eventually were identified as hazardous and subsequently controlled and monitored in nurses and pharmacists.

In the 1980s, we had no idea about the risks of exposure. We were just naïve young nurses impassioned about our careers, doing what needed to be done. My colleague laughed when doxorubicin inadvertently squirted out when she was priming the syringe, dotting the ceiling of the clean utility room with red splotches. A few years later, as graduate students, we read about the higher incidence of miscarriages in cancer nurses. Some friends of mine who were pregnant or trying to conceive opted out of administering chemotherapy when they could. Three decades later, new and larger studies would confirm the risks, reporting that nurses who handle chemotherapy drugs are twice as likely to have a miscarriage as colleagues who don't. As they age, these nurses also are more likely to get blood cancers or have nervous system and reproductive problems.

In 1986, NIOSH issued voluntary guidelines for safe handling of toxic drugs, and pharmacists began mixing chemotherapy under laminar air flow hoods, a vented workspace designed to protect the products from contamination as well as to shield the practitioner from breathing the vapors. The clinical guidelines were not mandatory, however, and donning gowns and gloves and masks consumed precious nursing time and cost. Patients get carefully calculated doses to treat their cancer; nurses get immeasurable exposure over years.

* * *

It took me longer to accept the fact that my exposure to chromium 51, a radioactive isotope, was potentially my most carcinogenic exposure. I initially denied its relative role in silent defense of my career.

In my doctoral program, I had chosen to study how the immune system responded to imagery and meditation in patients with cancer, which required using chromium in the laboratory to measure how well my patients' natural killer cells killed tumors in cell culture. Chromium is a gamma ray, the most penetrating ionizing radiation, that can damage DNA and cause cell death. It was the most sensitive test at the time. For a short time I also measured T-cell activity using tridiated thymidine, another radioisotope that isn't often used anymore. I trained in the techniques three years before I became pregnant with Brennan. Then later, when I was pregnant with Tyler, I continued to include the chromium assay in my own laboratory (using appropriate radioactive precautions).

The first day I trained in the lab, three years before becoming pregnant, Nancy, the technician who was mentoring me, introduced me to another female lab technician. Nancy commented as we walked away, "She has a two-year-old son with leukemia." Nancy said it without emotion, but she knew what it meant. Her daughter Betsy had died of leukemia years earlier, at the age of ten, following a relapse of ALL. Nancy talked about Betsy off and on over the years, but she said nothing more about the synchronicity of three mothers in the same lab having three children with leukemia. Neither did I.

* * *

I told Sara about the pesticides, chemotherapy, and radiation exposure, but I don't remember telling her about the ridiculous electromagnetic exposure at the airport just after Brennan's conception, when the screening gate agents made me go through the newly opened entrance gate to the gold concourse over and over again, each time removing another item of clothing or jewelry. "It must be set too sensitive," one of the young men said as I stripped down even more and walked through for the eighth time. Finally, they let me go on to my flight. I didn't think much about it at the time, but when I found out a few weeks later that I was pregnant, and I calculated that the day of my flight had been day eighteen of my menstrual cycle, I felt concerned.

There isn't any evidence that magnetic metal detectors trigger genetic translocations, although there is ongoing controversy over the association of electromagnetic frequencies and childhood leukemia. Exposure to atmospheric ionizing radiation while flying at high altitudes is probably more dangerous. There is a significant correlation between natural gamma rays and childhood leukemia. The new backscatter machines, initiated in some airports in 2009, use low-level ionizing radiation, which raises health concerns over cumulative exposure, even if each exposure is only ten microrems of radiation. Considering that a fetus is most susceptible to the teratogenic effects of ionizing radiation between two and fifteen weeks of gestation, and it was too late to change anything, I really didn't worry much more about the electromagnetic exposure. I had to cancel my next flight because I was in the hospital throwing up from the pregnancy.

Between my exposure to chlorpyrifos and the diagnosis of Brennan's leukemia seventeen years later, childhood cancer rates increased 1 percent per year. Something had to explain the rising incidence. Environmental exposures have long been suspected of causing childhood cancer, but the specific triggers have been difficult to identify, in part because cancer in children is rare and because each type of cancer may have different triggers. Despite the push for green environmental approaches, our society is increasingly exposed to gamma radiation, pesticides, diesel fuels, manufactured chemicals, and airborne particulate matter. We are more mobile and yet also more contained in our chemical-laden environments.

We also were older parents, although we snuck both boys in before we turned forty. The risk of childhood leukemia is reportedly 30 percent higher when mothers are thirty to forty years of age and even higher if they are over forty. Fathers offer a similar, age-related risk. The older we get, the greater the risk of cancer, for ourselves and our delayed offspring. In a recent study investigating autism rates, a child born to a twenty-year-old father had twenty-five mutations, compared to sixty-five mutations in a child born to a forty-year-old father. Mothers contributed fewer (fifteen) mutations, regardless of age. Although cancer originates in cells other than the sperm and egg, these mutations confirm what other studies have told us: older parental age contributes to chromosomal fragility, and chromosome breaks prime cells for cancer and other disorders. Telomeres, the protective protein at the ends of chromosomes, stabilize cells, but they shorten each time the cell divides, which is why they are markers of aging. Environmental toxins, inflammation, and stress also shorten telomeres.

Ultimately, cancer likely occurs in response to environmental exposures, gene mutations, *and* a faulty immune system. It is the environmental exposures that we can control.

* * *

As the list of exposures grew in my mind, I realized that I was starting to worry about everything, even things that seemed disproportionate to the risk.

"X-rays Triple Cancer Risk in Children," read a recent headline, referring to the increased incidence of leukemia and brain cancer in children who have more than five CT scans in their early years. Then there was "Gamma Rays Linked to Child Leukemia," implicating higher exposure to radioactive isotopes in soil, rocks, and drinking water. Yes, radiation triggers chromosomal breaks, and too much of anything, except vegetables, is never good. Later headlines trumpeted "Flu May Trigger Childhood Leukemia," "Insecticides: Potential Leukemia Risk," and "Child Leukemia Again Linked to Power Lines." Although I knew that these studies were correlational and couldn't imply causation, the boys would get mercury-free flu shots, and we would avoid pesticides and chemicals as much as feasible (even when lice nested in Tyler's shoulder-length, thick, curly hair).

I also decided to contact a lawyer to spur the power company to bury the power line that had draped over our roof for six years. It wasn't a high-voltage power line, but it still represented a consistent daily dose of electromagnetic exposure. The power line entered the electrical box on the outside wall of the living room, in the corner where Brennan spent hours every day drawing and designing at his kid-size table. To get to the power box from the neighborhood transformer, the cable had to drape over the roof, just above the window seat where I had placed Tyler in his bassinet every morning to gather sunlight to counteract his newborn jaundice. Even the cat regularly slept there. And he died of cancer.

Some studies have found no relationship between electromagnetic exposure and childhood leukemia. Most of these studies tested exposure levels in the middle of the rooms, not in the corners where children sat at their tables. Other studies found a relatively weak link, attributing the effect to altered signals that regulate normal cell growth. After Brennan's diagnosis, I bought a handheld EMF reader and found that the electromagnetic levels were ten times higher in that corner of the living room, closer to the outside electrical box, than they were in the middle of the room.

The "hot dog scare" surfaced when Brennan was about three years old, before diagnosis. "Hotdogs Increase Leukemia Risk in Children!" the headlines shouted. The study they cited had found that 232 children with leukemia who had eaten more than twelve hot dogs per month had nine times the normal risk of developing childhood leukemia when compared to a matched control group without leukemia. A child whose dad ate twelve or more hot dogs per month also was at higher risk. I had to wonder: Does anyone, other than someone with season tickets to their local baseball team or someone gorging in an eating competition, really eat that many hot dogs?

To its credit, the study factored in the protective effects of Vitamin C and controlled for other environmental risk factors that the children were exposed to. Regardless, a higher than expected consumption incriminated the standard grocery store hot dog, the one with nitrites added as a preservative and coloring agent. Because the study used a correlational design, however, it couldn't conclude that hotdogs *caused* leukemia; it could only acknowledge that children who ate a lot of hot dogs also were at greater risk for leukemia. And it wasn't just hot dogs, it was all deli meats, as well as bacon with nitrites.

Nothing more ever came of the hot dog study, but additional studies with children have confirmed the association of cancer with nitrites, and studies in rats have implicated a causative effect of nitrites on tumor growth. The dose remains important. The more you eat, the greater the risk.

At the time, I felt pretty safe about any actual hot dog risk, as I rarely let Brennan eat them. If he did, they were the nitrite-free-hormone-free-all-natural-beef-grass-fed hot dogs from the local co-op. I had already banned many of these additives from our home because of my own chemical-free food sensitivity diet. Brennan ate commercial hot dogs at baseball games and birthday parties, and that was about it.

For whatever reason, I needed to explore the avenues of my son's illness. Asking *why* Brennan had gotten leukemia allowed me to better understand the circumstances. I couldn't change the past and I couldn't control every exposure, but I could make some sense of their impact on our lives.

According to attribution theory, individuals have a strong need to understand events by attributing some cause for them. If it's human nature, then other parents must question too, and I am not alone in wondering why.

* * *

After Brennan's diagnosis, I feared for Tyler's safety. Other than the key fact that his was a different pregnancy, Tyler had been exposed to the same environment and possessed the same immune predisposition. And he'd had two CT scans of his head by age five because of recurrent headaches and a concussion from a fall on the ice. A family I would meet on a pediatric listserv had two boys diagnosed with leukemia, one year apart. The fear that Tyler too could succumb to leukemia would haunt me until he turned four and a half, and then five, and six, and continued on, although to a lesser degree, until he reached his teens. Every year on his birthday I would breathe a sigh of relief and say a prayer of gratitude. Teenagers get leukemia too, but T-cell ALL is more common—and according to Mel Greaves, the TEL-AML1 fusion has a limited lifespan effect of approximately ten years.

I was determined to protect both my boys from as many environmental toxins and exposures as I could, without isolating them (too much!) from friends and normal childhood experiences. Tyler would start preschool and Brennan would go to kindergarten during his first year of treatment. They would be exposed to other children, which would be a good thing for Tyler's developing immune system but a greater risk for Brennan, whose immune system was suppressed from daily chemotherapy. And, of course, I would catch everything they did. Life would remain a precarious balance and a blur. For three years I would whoosh through the days, assessing and controlling risks and holding my breath through every symptom and illness.

Once Brennan passed the relapse risk and Tyler was well past the peak incidence age, I would realize that there was only so much I could control or was willing to change. We made choices as parents. I wasn't willing to move from the city to avoid the exhaust from the adjoining highway or the power plant less than a mile away. None of our neighbors had cancer. I wasn't going to prevent our children from playing in parks and swimming at the pool or beach. The rigors and precautions surrounding Brennan's treatment were already isolating enough. And I wasn't yet ready to abandon my career, which included laboratory work with chromium.

What I could do was to continue serving organic food and avoiding chemicals and pesticides at home. It wouldn't be foolproof, however. And although I would work hard to cook every meal from raw and natural ingredients, Brennan's intense cravings while on treatment meant his menu was often replete with processed cheese and even hot dogs (nitrite-free, of course). Reversing three years of this high-fat, salt-laden diet would take immense patience and compromise after his treatment ended.

* * *

When Brennan was diagnosed, I couldn't think beyond my exposures and our situation. I couldn't even consider Sara's unborn baby. I was focused solely on making sense of the events in our lives. Now, sitting next to Sara, I had traced my exposure to radiation, chemicals, and viruses, the known triggers for gene translocations and immune dysfunction, even though I had no idea if and how they could affect a fetus up to a decade later.

As I talked, Sara just nodded her head, not in any sort of confirmation of my thoughts, but in acknowledgment of my need to say them. I think I knew that I never would have an answer. But there it was, evidence exposed and opened up like a tulip, inviting us to examine it at will. And Sara just listened, either because she knew what I needed and was willing to just be there for me or because she was a caring, empathetic nurse. At that moment, I didn't need someone countering my thoughts, asking me questions, or questioning my information or assumptions. I needed time to figure things out for myself. All parents deserve such a blessing.

CHAPTER 10

Surviving

The first two months of treatment are among the most intense phases in the leukemia protocols. We had achieved remission, and now our February mission was to secure, or "consolidate," the induction, with a primary focus on preventing cells from hiding out in the central nervous system. This was the only month in three years of treatment that required weekly intrathecal chemotherapy.

Once every week, Brennan would have to face the dreaded back medicine and swirling tornado of white anesthetic. He also had to be NPO—nothing by mouth—the night before and the morning of treatment. I expected him to rebel, considering that he'd started the month with ten days of high-dose prednisone, a steroid that made him feel as if he could both be a grizzly bear and eat one. But he didn't complain. He just did what was expected of him.

On good days, Brennan and Tyler raced around the "Indy Loop" on their scooters, wearing a path over the new hardwood floors, calling out, "Time me, Mom!" as they sped past the kitchen clock. I can still see the floor markings where they leaned left, dragging their suede-slippered feet to keep their balance around the corners, Brennan always in the lead.

I have video clips of them competing in long-distance jumps from the living room couch. They tossed the cushions off as far as they could and then, balancing on the wobbly springs, feet apart and arms twirling, they leaped onto the cushions strewn out like stepping stones on the floor. Then they ran laps over the cushions and around the couch, singing "Row, Row, Row Your Boat" and other silly songs. Some nights they channeled Buzz Lightyear, exclaiming, "To infinity and beyond!" as they synchronized their leaps off the family room window seat and onto the two parallel leather couches, sliding across on their tummies, giggling as they jumped up to do it again.

Duane had started traveling again after deciding to take a new job "for security." At first I thought he meant financial security, but since I carried our family's health insurance that provided excellent coverage, I could only imagine that working was *his* security, giving him meaning and purpose and control over something. After all, work was what he knew best. He had something he was interested in, it would help out a friend (who recruited him), and he had already made up his mind. But the job required a fair amount of travel, which left me alone many weekday evenings, and I scrambled to find a sitter for the evenings I taught.

On nights when Duane was home, the boys shot Nerf balls into the basketball hoop hoisted high on the French doors of the living room. Duane rebounded while I clocked the seconds, shot video, and cheered. It was a relief not to have to orchestrate activities.

To refuel, Brennan ate at least every two hours. In one day, he consumed nine homemade, plate-size chicken, rice, and cheese burritos. The steroids had hijacked his pituitary's satiety mechanism. It's no wonder constipation and gastrointestinal obstructions were common side effects of this phase of treatment.

When exhausted, he crashed, but only when his tummy was full and he could no longer force his body to move and his mind to create, always after ten p.m. Then he'd be up by 5 a.m., ready to play cribbage golf and other board games on the living room floor with Duane, the other early riser. Tyler kept up as best he could, napping in between activities.

On the weekends, Duane and I tag-teamed, squeezing in grocery and pharmacy stops with caffeine to go from the coffee shop. On Sunday nights, Duane and I would sigh and admit TGIM to each other: "Thank God it's Monday and we can go back to work tomorrow."

On more challenging days, verbal crusades replaced activities and games.

"No, I'm *not* going with you. You can take Tyler; Dad can stay home with me."

"But I can't sleep! I've tried counting sheep and singing songs and reading stories. Can you play a game with me in bed?"

"But you *have* to, I *need* you to—right now! I can't wait for you to give Tyler a bath! And no, I won't take one with him. He takes up too much room. I need the whole tub!"

"But I'm *starving*! I need to eat right *now*! I can't wait!"

By the third week of consolidation, we all started to unravel.

Brennan would work himself into a frenzy, insisting and demanding, until he eventually melted down physically. Sometimes the back-and-forth negotiations consumed an hour or more, simply because "I'm done with this conversation" or "Stop! We are not discussing this anymore" didn't register in his persistent determination. Full of adrenaline-induced strength, he fought me off like a fire-breathing dragon. He was too feisty for me to pick up and carry, although Duane could and still would.

On occasion, after a particularly challenging encounter, Duane would get Brennan calmed and then come to me, lying exhausted or reading student papers in bed, and ask, "What should I do?"

My compassion, as empty as the water in the well, would allow me only to shrug my shoulders and say, "I don't know"—thinking all the while that if I did know what to do, I would have done it myself. And "doing" something wasn't the answer, anyway. Over years of parenting, I would highlight passages from parenting advice books, leaving him a note to "read this" for perspective. I'm pretty sure he ignored most of them, probably because the crisis of the moment had passed. Parenting a child with leukemia requires limitless strength, ingenuity, patience, and stamina—and help. I can't imagine how single parents survive.

Sometimes I would call my twin brother Jerry and ask for his advice. He didn't have children, and he taught young adults in college, but Brennan had seemingly inherited his determination and ingenuity and persistence, and I expected Jerry to have some insight. Both Jerry and Brennan were "out-of-the-box" thinkers, and I often needed fresh perspective. My brother always offered advice, and he would follow our conversations with an e-mail offering new suggestions or strategies, contemplated after we got off the phone. What I came to value most, however, was his nonjudgmental, listening ear and his compassionate desire to help. Just knowing that he was available and willing to listen and help me process gave me strength to keep trying.

* * *

Brennan's strength eventually overpowered mine. One night he yanked his bedroom door open as I stood bracing it shut, trying to enforce a non-interactive time out in his room. Admitting defeat, I simply turned my back on him and opened the next nearest door, the kids' bathroom. Following a series of house renovations, it just happened to be the only original door in the house with a functioning lock. I locked myself in.

Once in solitude, I sat on the closed toilet stool, staring at the white and celadon tile framing the narrow room with the slanted ceiling, built as a dormer into the roof of the house. It was cozy. But it was a bathroom. I had given myself the time out. As I wondered what to do and how long to stay in this confined space, I thought through the potential consequences of leaving a not-yet five- and two-year-old free to their own devices. Tyler was in his crib and Brennan was screaming outside the door, "Mom! I need you! Mom! Listen to me!"

I deemed them safe, for the moment, anyway. I knew that Brennan just wanted to drag me back into the verbal volleyball that would ultimately lead to his win. With Mercury ruling his Gemini planet, talking was his forte, and he could go on for hours. With only slight hesitation, I took off my clothes and stepped into the tub. I sucked in a quick breath as the almost scalding shower stream pelted my frazzled and fragile psyche. I needed the shower to hurt, to wake me up, to make me see the reality of my dysfunction. Or I just needed the shower to take control.

I emerged calm and centered, but not exactly with a plan of what to do next. It was quiet. Too quiet. As I toweled off and got dressed, I spotted a jagged, torn corner of white construction paper on the floor, that had been slipped under the door. Brennan had scrawled in large block print in blue marker, "Mom. I calmed down. Please listen to me."

The maturity of his writing and message didn't register with me right away. I wouldn't trust my memory if I hadn't saved the scrap of paper. I cautiously but confidently opened the door, not sure what to expect. He had left the door to his bedroom open and I found him curled up in bed, lying on his side, facing me, waiting.

I sighed, feeling restored and more supportive. Now we could talk.

I understood the power of prednisone to drive his fractious energy, and I tried to be patient with the physical aggression and lashing out. After all, I had been there myself, under the influence of weeks of high-dose prednisone for slow-to-respond asthma. I knew what it felt like to feel out of control of one's emotions and motivations. Those were times I was best left alone to my idiosyncratic tendencies, to withdraw and crank out thirty-page book chapters in a weekend or clean out every closet in the house, whether it needed it or not. Later, I would wonder what happened to that favorite sweater or spare sheet set, and I often didn't recognize my writing when it came back in galley form months after. I'm still embarrassed by the time I spouted off to the statistician on a ten-person conference call, announcing, "We lost our window. The time to do that was six months ago, but we didn't have the data then." The prednisone-induced frenzied energy sparked whatever thought that flitted into my head to burst out uncensored. It didn't seem to matter that I struggled with every breath and could barely walk up one flight of stairs. My mind compensated for the physical paralysis, stimulated by random ideas and superfluous thoughts that I convinced myself needed action, immediately. I would finally crash after weeks of three to four hours of sleep a night. Everything just felt so out of control.

I tried to be more sympathetic when I realized that Brennan's little body, one-third the size of mine, was captive to the same dose of extra cortisol, triggering his already active alert brain and restless muscles. *He isn't trying to be challenging,* I reminded myself each time he lashed out at me physically or corralled his toddler brother in the chair, demanding that he do his bidding. Although he seemed aware of his dramatic responses, he was unable to calm himself. And he certainly wasn't going to allow me to calm him.

But drawing did. One day during this tumultuous time, he sketched a self-portrait. Heavily outlined in dark blue, black, and purple, his face was again topped with a mound of hair. Purple accents on his hips, arms, and prominent tongue bellowing in a wide-open mouth seemed to shout stubbornness and defiance. I labeled the picture "an angry day."

Brennan's emotional outbursts seemed to mirror his physical symptoms, and over time I deduced that they forecasted impending illness. He consistently acted out the day before he became symptomatic of a cold, ear infection, or strep throat. "Maybe he's getting sick," I speculated when he regressed emotionally. I didn't track my predictability rate, but it was accurate more often than not, which reinforced my vigilance. I started to anticipate the storms.

After one particularly long weekend, I called Sara, Brennan's nurse. I had tried writing in my journal, hoping for insight. *Why is he acting out and resisting so? Why is he so verbally loud and abusive? Why does he need so much control this week in particular?*

"Sara, I need your help," I pleaded into the phone.

"What's going on?" she responded in her calm and reassuring voice, the one I really needed to hear at that moment.

"Brennan acted out all weekend. He fought back on everything." I told her about his physical aggression and then reminded her that he'd had his fourth weekly intrathecal chemotherapy on Thursday and a 101.5-degree fever on Friday. His counts had bounced up and down over the past ten days, with abnormal levels of absolute neutrophil counts of 6,000 to 600 to 14,000.

"Could something physical explain this behavior?" I asked.

"Yes, it might be the intrathecal," she said.

After talking to Brennan's doctor, she called back. "Yes, Dr. Steve thinks it is arachnoiditis, inflammation of the lining of the spinal cord. This can happen with intrathecal, especially after four weeks in a row. We could add more prednisone."

I cringed. After talking through the pros and cons, we decided to just wait it out.

I found out later that this first clinical trial with "triples" caused seizures and strokes in some children, convincing the research group to drop the triple combination from future clinical trials. I was relieved that Brennan hadn't experienced these severe neurological reactions, and I felt compassion and concern for the parents whose children had. I still wondered, though, about the long-term neurotoxic effect of triples. It would take decades to really know. At the moment, I was just relieved to have an explanation for his out-bursts.

I created a bedtime chart, and I spent more time talking to Brennan, asking about his reactions, how he was feeling. I listened. By letting go of trying to figure things out, shedding my responsible and analytical role, I could focus on getting him, and us, through that trying time. It was such a relief to just be Mom.

* * *

We were in survival mode, where protective instincts prevailed and perspectives got distorted. I didn't really think about how to balance all of my roles. I raced home every day from work or the clinic to cook dinner, give meds, make snacks, read books, and, after the boys were asleep, grade papers, read my students' thesis drafts, or dig up literature for my next lecture. As a cancer nurse, educator, researcher, and mom, I naturally assumed responsibility. I was the most prepared of anyone.

Eventually, the acute stress of surviving evolved into chronic stress of imbalance. The demands accumulated, and the only thing I cut back on were weekend hours at the office. On the afternoon that we arrived home from the hospital that first week, I had answered the phone and spontaneously agreed to do NIH (National Institutes of Health) grant reviews. Now, two months later, after getting through consolidation and submitting winter quarter grades, I sat facing the box of eight grants in a state of total exhaustion.

I had said "yes" at a vulnerable time. I didn't know what the next day would bring, much less the coming months. Before answering, I had hesitated, aware of this uncertainty. In retrospect, I should have trusted my gut and said "no." I didn't even think to tell the administrator that my son had leukemia. I didn't need an excuse if it was something I wanted to do. Being asked to review was an honor; it meant that my own research was respected. I had waited for this opportunity. But I wasn't prepared for the monstrosity of the task in the midst of adrenal exhaustion.

It would be eight more years before I would start treatment for adrenal insufficiency. But even in those early months of my son's treatment, I had started to see the recurring pattern of mind numbing

and physically exhausting, can-barely-get-out-of-bed fatigue sur-
facing after major stressors and then taking weeks to resolve. I was
exhausted, drained, and weak, and I could barely concentrate, much
less read, interpret, and write a critique for more than one grant per
day. I had pushed my body to its maximum for two months and it
desperately needed a break. It was spring break for the students, but
I couldn't stop. I had said yes.

I forced myself to tackle the grant reviews at work during the
day and to take them home in the evenings. It took me four days to
complete two reviews. It was Friday, I had six left, and spring quarter
started on Monday. I was so exhausted I was almost in tears. I called
a colleague who reviewed regularly for NIH, and I asked for her
advice. She immediately dropped what she was doing and ran down
from her office, one floor above mine, to be with me in my dilemma.

"What can I do, Cheryl?" I pleaded. "I can't finish these. It's just
not possible."

After discussing the options, she gave me the permission I
needed to admit defeat. It was my first lesson in letting go.

"Call her back and tell her you can't do them," she said. "Ship
them back."

"Can I really do that?" I asked. Having never reviewed before, I
wasn't familiar with the process or the expectations.

"It has to be," Cheryl said.

I rarely, if ever, gave up on anything. I honored my commitments
and often over-extended myself reaching them. To compensate, I
just worked harder. But at the time, I couldn't possibly do what I had
asked my body to do. I could barely hold my head up without my
hands for support.

I had tested stress-hormone-immune relationships in my
research. When stress is short-term or mild, cortisol levels increase
and then return to normal when the challenge is over. But over time,
when stress becomes chronic and continuous, such as in a constant
hypervigilant state, cortisol remains high. Eventually, the adrenal
glands either stop responding to the hypothalamic-pituitary-adrenal
(HPA) axis trigger in the brain or the pituitary stops produc-
ing hormones that trigger the adrenals. In my recurring state of
over-extension, I had depleted the cortisol that got me up in the

morning and prompted my muscles to move and my brain to process. I felt like I was pushing a doorbell repeatedly, expecting someone to be there, and no one was answering. Even though surviving meant "doing," I had to learn to stop doing in order to survive.

When I called the grants administrator back, the conversation went something like this:

"I am really sorry, but I just can't complete the reviews. I finished the two primary reviews, but I just can't do the other six, the ones that I am a secondary or tertiary reviewer on. Is there someone else you can give them to?"

"You have ten more days before the review session," she said. "You could send your scores in a little late."

"Thank you, but I absolutely cannot do them. I am too ill to complete them. And I only have four more days before the new term starts."

"Well, then, do them in four days and send them in."

"Tricia, you aren't listening to me!" I blurted, and then slowly enunciated, "I cannot do these reviews. I am sending them back to you."

After a long pause, during which I felt even more adamant and confident about my decision to let the reviews go, she replied, "Hold on to them until I can find out where to ship them."

"Thank you," I said, exhaling with mixed relief and exasperation, and we hung up without another word. The next day I received directions to send the box to a gracious reviewer in Indiana.

I would never again be asked to review for that particular institute, although I would review for a different NIH study section after Brennan came off treatment.

After that first experience, I adopted a twenty-four-hour rule. I could not say "yes" to a request unless I had twenty-four hours to think it over. I don't think I have ever regretted a delayed decision, but I have, many times, regretted saying "yes" on the spur of the moment. I always wanted to help when needed.

* * *

During this time of intense existence, Brennan drew an abstract picture of his bones. "The green cells are the brain and the red inside is the heart," he told me. He knew that a heart and brain were vital to life, and they would help him survive leukemia. He reminded me that I, too, needed both.

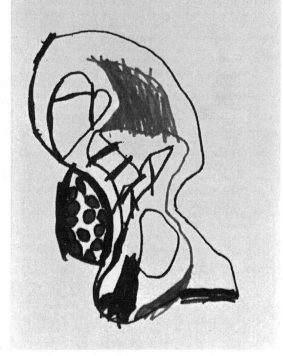

Brennan's bones.

CHAPTER 11

I Just Want to Live in the Moment

March arrived, along with our first Interim Maintenance, offering a reprieve from the intense chemo schedule. Brennan drew his first sailboat. It had a hefty, walnut-shaped, dark blue hull with two red sails sitting on top. It sat alone in the midst of deep, dark water. In the left corner of the light gray sky, he had printed vertically down the side, one word per line, "Brennan, Love Mom, Love Dad, Love Tyler." I smiled, noting Tyler's presence back in his brother's worldview. He might feel alone out there on the water, but at least he'd brought his family with him.

Until he drew this picture, I didn't know that Brennan cared or knew anything about sailing. Duane and I had taken sailing lessons in Boston Harbor the year the tall ships had anchored in the bay. Had we talked about dodging them in our efforts to stay afloat and out of trouble as we tried to catch the wind in the swift, twenty-foot soling? We sailed a few times on Lake Michigan in Chicago, but we hadn't sailed since moving to Minnesota.

Brennan didn't always show me his pictures. I discovered this one in the notebook he started drawing in while at the hospital. The thin paper sometimes bled through to other pictures, as this one did. It was the only paper I had with me at the time.

"That's where I want to be," I said softly to myself as I sat down in the living room with the notebook after Brennan had gone to bed. "I want to sit in the middle of that ocean, bobbing up and down along with the rhythm of the waves." I let out a long sigh. I was so relieved to have a break in the intensity of treatment. I knew that eventually

I would have to hoist the sails and turn the boat downwind and get back to doing what needed to be done. For the moment, however, I just wanted to be.

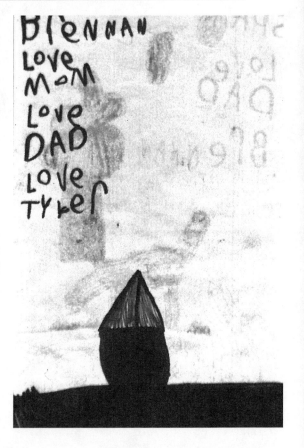

* * *

We had survived induction and consolidation. I felt an immense sense of relief. Some families never get that far. Still, we had three more years of treatment to go.

Sara and I reviewed the new Interim Maintenance (IM) road map together.

Brennan's sailboat—sailing alone.

"He gets prednisone starting today," she said, "the 6-TG every day, and the methotrexate once a week. Just come back in two weeks to check counts."

"Two weeks?" I asked. "You mean we don't have to come into the clinic for two weeks?"

I took in a deep, anticipatory breath, filling my lungs with hope. It was like coming up for air after being submerged underwater with your eyes closed. The sky looked bluer, the day brighter. Even the road map looked less cluttered, less frantic. *I can pace myself,* I thought. I could actually envision the entire month ahead, without being overwhelmed by each individual day. And I knew what to expect. The familiar brought a new sense of security.

Over the next twenty-eight days, Brennan would continue to take oral chemotherapy every day at home, but he wouldn't have to get any, *any*, intravenous, intrathecal, or intramuscular shots for an entire twenty-eight days. Reveling in the freedom, I danced to the parking lot.

* * *

The relief was short-lived. Three days later Brennan had an ear infection and we were back in the clinic. Two weeks later his counts bottomed out, necessitating his first dose reduction in oral chemotherapy. Thankfully, he didn't have to get any intravenous infusions.

Dose reductions from that day forward would no longer be made up. Like school closing "grace" days in a snowy winter, we would no longer extend treatment because of missed or lowered doses. While the certainty of the fixed end-date, March 6, 2000, reaffirmed that leukemia was a journey with an outcome, three years would take us into the next millennium!

I knew that too many dose reductions could increase the risk for relapse and reduce chances for survival, but I kept my son out of the equation as much as I could, preferring to envision the treatment decisions as numbers on the page. Brennan had survived the first two months, when about 5 percent of kids don't. It was a delicate balance of treating for cure and managing side effects. I let his medical team track the setbacks and worry about the dose reductions as we inched our way through the month.

* * *

I liked this new schedule. By early April, we were halfway through IM, and I expected to savor the emerging spring, budding trees, and extra hours of light after an exceptionally frigid Minnesota winter. Laurie and I stood outside together, enjoying the gentle, warming sun on our faces, as Brennan climbed into his car seat, ready to head to the clinic to start the second twenty-eight-day cycle of Interim Maintenance #1.

"I can't believe we are standing outside in the sunshine, in the exact same place I was packing up the car to go to the hospital three months ago," I said to Laurie. "It seems so long ago. I am so looking forward to this next month."

* * *

The second twenty-eight-day launch of IM#1 should have gone like the first. We would check in at the clinic, Brennan would beat me at PacMan until someone called us to measure his height and weight, then Sara would draw his blood from his port-a-cath and send it off for "counts" while Brennan and I read books together and played Nerf basketball in the treatment room.

When his counts came back, Sara would give him the intravenous vincristine, the only chemotherapy scheduled for that day, and we would go home where he would take his dish of pills after dinner. It was the exact same treatment as the last twenty-eight days.

But nothing was predictable in this new world.

One of the oncologists we didn't see regularly walked in to examine Brennan before he got his chemotherapy. She turned to look at me, stethoscope in her ears, as she lifted the back of Brennan's shirt to listen to his lungs. "Next month when you come in, you will start the first delayed intensification," she said as she listened to his lungs in between her own breaths.

I stood against the wall with crossed arms.

"Take another deep breath, Brennan," she said as she continued talking, apparently to me. "It's the hardest of all the treatment phases. We see the most complications during DI. Things like pneumonia, aseptic necrosis of the joints, and infections. He might need a blood transfusion."

She kept going, reminding me that we would be in clinic three days a week and that hospitalization was likely during that eight week "re-induction" period.

I should have interjected, "STOP!" or, at least, "Wait a minute, please," but I didn't. My mind screamed for time to sort out the confusion of why she was telling me this now, twenty-eight days before I needed to hear it. I was furious, but also unsettled. I respected this doctor; I knew she knew better than I did what DI was like. But how was this early warning benefiting us? She had jumped right over these next twenty-eight days, the ones that I so wanted to savor, to enjoy, to appreciate. I wanted to cling to the moment, and she was yanking me forward.

We silently walked out of the clinic, the treatment bag bumping against my right leg with every step, Brennan sidled up to the other. I had gone in for the appointment optimistic and hopeful. I wanted and desperately needed to live for that day. I wanted to feel the reward of making it that far.

* * *

Laurie was sitting at the kitchen table as we walked in the door at home. "How did it go?" she asked cheerfully.

Brennan went off to find Tyler, and I scorched out my response. "How dare she prepare us for what is to come twenty-eight days later!" I filled her in, and she nodded sympathetically.

"How did Brennan take it?" Laurie asked.

I stared back with a blank look, then, thankful for her reminder, I went off to find Brennan. I located him in the family room, immersed in driving cars through the carwash ramp with his brother. I let him play.

* * *

As a graduate student, years before Brennan's birth, I had a patient who taught me the value of first assessing where the patient is at. On her second visit to the clinic, I approached Mrs. M in the waiting room and sat down in the chair next to her. She came alone, as she did through most of her treatments. She wore a navy jacket and pants and sat stiffly, looking straight ahead, her hands folded in her lap over her purse.

I sat down next to Mrs. M and asked how she was. I then launched into my agenda. At least, that's what I remember. I needed to obtain her written consent for treatment. She had to know what to expect when she went into the hospital that day for her first chemotherapy to treat her non–Hodgkin's lymphoma. Papers in hand, I promptly went over the complete list of side effects and self-assuredly suggested how she should prepare for her two days in the hospital. She would have to wake up every four hours to take leucovorin, a specific medication that would "rescue" her normal cells from dying after the high doses of methotrexate. The cancer cells wouldn't take up the rescue drug, but the normal cells would. If she missed doses, her counts could bottom out and she could become critically ill. I talked on, acutely aware of the need to have my patient fully informed before consenting to treatment. I worked hard to remember everything I needed to say. I might even have practiced the night before.

In the middle of my litany, Mrs. M stood up and walked through the door, out of the clinic, and into the hall without looking back.

I froze, my breath shallow. My mind raced over the "teaching" I had forced upon her, the rapid speech I often used, the unfamiliar terms sprinkled on the page. I then imagined myself in her shoes, sighed at my realization, and got up and slowly approached as she shuffled around in the hallway. I was relieved that she didn't back away from me.

"Mrs. M, I am so sorry. This must be too much information, too fast." I paused, and when she didn't say anything, I added, "What is it that you need right now?"

She looked around, avoiding my eyes. She paced a bit and then said in a shaky voice, "I don't know. It's just so overwhelming."

"Maybe if we take it slower. Let's get a cup of tea and go over what you need to know for tonight. We'll take it one step at a time. I'll come see you in the hospital tomorrow."

She nodded, her lips pursed together, and we walked back into the clinic.

I still smile now, three decades later, when I think of Mrs. M. She taught me to consider and respect what a patient needs and to individualize and adapt my approach. Only after slowing down could I focus on being present in that moment with her. She clearly communicated her needs, even though she wasn't able to verbalize them. Had she not walked out of that room, I might never have given her a chance to tell me.

After that day, we worked together in a supportive and warm relationship throughout her treatment. I worked at asking and listening, rather than telling. And she worked at telling me what she wanted and needed in any given moment. I learned that information is only useful if it is received.

As Mrs. M sat on her bed during her second hospitalization, I said, "Remember, you have to take the leucovorin every four hours throughout the night. The nurses will wake you up."

"I want to do it myself," she said, raising her eyes to mine.

"Okay. What will work for you?"

We talked over the possible options to allow her more independence.

Finally, I said, "I'll get you an alarm clock this afternoon, and you can set it every four hours."

And that's what worked for the remainder of her treatments. She never missed a dose.

* * *

Fifteen years later, when it was Brennan and me being bombarded with the agenda, it was my turn to advocate for myself. But instead of standing up, as Mrs. M had, I had retreated, dragging along the fears and anxieties I was trying so hard to let go of for twenty-eight days. Instead of living in the moment, being present to myself, I had let that moment consume me.

If I wanted to stay centered, I had to resist taking on the agenda of the healthcare team. It wasn't intentional, but acting as both a mother and a nurse meant that I was always looking out for someone else. If I wanted to be an effective advocate for my family, and myself, I had to become aware of my own needs and learn to communicate them, as Mrs. M had.

Many years later, I would understand what my nursing friends meant when they repeatedly advised me, "Take care of yourself." I always thought taking care of *me* would require extra time—an extra hour or two for a massage or reading or self-indulgence—that I didn't have or couldn't allow myself. Things would just pile up in my absence. I would eventually see how simply thinking about my own needs and advocating for myself could protect and nourish my well-being. Taking care of me required a mind shift, not a time shift. I needed to learn how to respond to situations from a center of stillness and calm, as if I were on that boat in the middle of the ocean, balancing the boat *and* directing our course.

The unexpected winds kept tossing me around. Laurie submitted her resignation that month. She didn't want to be Brennan's caregiver anymore. "I prefer to be his friend," she said, though she promised to stay through both of his DI treatments.

I don't know if this five-month warning was to see Brennan through DI, to give us more time to prepare, or to ensure a steady salary until she found a new job, but I understood Laurie's choice. Caregiving was her job. She hadn't signed up for this.

It was only later, after she left, that I wondered if I had been too busy or too distracted to notice her unhappiness. Had I ever asked her how she was doing, how she was feeling? It must have taken strength and courage to advocate for herself, her own needs. She was one step ahead of me.

When May arrived, I wasn't ready to hoist the sails, but I knew that our collective inner strength would stabilize the boat through conceivable storms.

CHAPTER 12

And How Is Mom?

"And how is Mom?" Dr. Dan asked as we settled into the clinic room for our first visit together. We sat in a powwow, Brennan on my left, Dr. Dan on my right. As a physician specializing in behavioral pediatrics and hypnosis, Dr. Dan knew how to help kids.

"Me?" I asked, incredulous that he would inquire about my well-being. After all, Brennan was the reason we were together that day. Five months into treatment, halfway through DI#1, Brennan and The Leukemia now reigned over our day-to-day life. We had become backseat drivers on the road map and the intense behavioral outbursts and uncompromising demands of a four-year-old on prednisone and decadron, steroids that were critical pulses of treatment. Without realizing it, we had relinquished the keys and put Brennan in the driver's seat.

It wasn't a totally unfamiliar role. Since birth, Brennan had known how to rev our engines in response to his intense internal drive and to steer our schedules to accommodate his enthusiastic energy and interests. Perhaps he was a typical first child, the one that redefines family life, but he seemed to have inherited an extra dose of "need for speed," and he had us trained by the time he was two. The problem was that he wanted to race that car, and I wanted to float on a boat.

No one felt in control. Brennan simply reacted to the energy overdrive of the medication and his natural survival mechanisms, and the rest of us tried to keep up. When he was wound up, he seemed unable to escape the intensity of the moment.

Serotonin, a calming neurotransmitter found in the gut and brain, falls during stressful situations, especially when the situation feels inescapable or uncontrollable. Low serotonin leaves a person feeling overwhelmed until he either shuts down from sadness or explodes with aggression. It's more complicated than that, but it helped me to understand that Brennan's responses were in part biochemical. I didn't know if he was reacting more to the emotional stress or to the steroids. I just knew that we both needed help in finding some calm in the midst of daily storms.

From my work, I knew that stress directly suppresses the immune system, reducing the ability of T cells and natural killer cells to fight cancer and viruses. That's why college students often get sick during or just after final exams. Stress also affects sleep, eating, and exercise habits, and it can actually destroy the dendrites of the hippocampus, where learning and memory take place. Over time, cortisol, secreted in response to stress, reprograms how the hypothalamic-pituitary-adrenal (HPA) axis responds, triggering hypervigilant or blunted responses. Children are even more susceptible than adults to the neurocognitive effects of excess cortisol.

We couldn't change the stressor, the cancer, so we had to learn to change our response.

At the time, I was just hoping that Dr. Dan could teach Brennan new skills to manage his stress. If Brennan could feel like he had some control over his responses, at least when prednisone wasn't driving his behavior, we might be happier at home. I didn't want this aggressive response pattern to become ingrained, like his altered eating habits ultimately did.

Of course, it wasn't just Brennan. I didn't realize it at the time, but my own frazzled energy was inextricably linked to his. It was just easier for me to see his actions rather than my own. We both were exhausted, acting and reacting, swinging like monkeys in trees.

I looked at Dr. Dan. "How am I?" I reflected back.

This was the first time since Brennan's diagnosis that someone, anyone, had asked *me* how I was doing. A wave of realization washed over me as I held my breath and my heart fluttered in my chest: I wasn't sure! I had never thought to check in with *me*, to ask myself how I was doing. Could he see the surprise on my face, the uncertainty?

"Okay. I'm doing okay. I think." I vowed to give it more thought.

In the years to come, post-traumatic stress disorder (PTSD) and post-traumatic stress symptoms (PTSS) would become common labels for anyone who has survived a life-threatening and traumatic event and is exhibiting intrusive thoughts, avoidance, or arousal. In the decade following Brennan's diagnosis, twenty studies would address these adjustment disorders in parents of childhood cancer survivors. Up to two-thirds of mothers and half of fathers had PTSS while their child was in treatment.

It is common for people with PTSD/PTSS to relive their distressing memories and go out of their way to avoid reminders. They either suppress their feelings until they are numb or feel excessive guilt and worry, staying on constant alert. They may have difficulty sleeping and concentrating. Some veterans of the Vietnam, Gulf, and Iraq wars have classic PTSD and are unable to function in their daily life. The rest of us probably have stress-related symptoms of varying degrees.

Not everyone exposed to the same event will get PTSD. Interestingly, veterans who have a brain injury in the amygdala do not get PTSD because they cannot re-induce fear related to the traumatic event. For most of us, managing our fear involves an intricate balance between being aware of it and interpreting its meaning in the moment. Is it surprising that seeking equilibrium between thinking and feeling drives behavior?

It's not easy to keep perspective when fear overpowers thinking. It's natural to avoid, or bury, what we cannot change, what we think we have no control over. I fought back tears those first few days when I called family on the phone from Brennan's hospital room. He didn't need the burden of my distress. And I was better at thinking than I was at feeling.

We were in our fifth month of treatment, and although the two-month delayed intensification was indeed intense, with new and aggressive treatment, I was better prepared. Recent studies in parents report that stress symptoms decrease after the first six months. *Check.* But the effects can linger. *Uh-oh.* The stress that some parents experience during treatment can predict how well they adjust after treatment ends. *But don't all parents feel stressed to the max?* I wondered. What about the families that were hospitalized more frequently, or had only one parent, no support at home, limited financial resources, or long distances to travel to treatment? Compared to people in those situations, we were fortunate. But perhaps it wasn't that the stress was greater for some families than others, but that the ability to adapt differed. Some parents might make better chameleons.

Stress is ubiquitous, but how we respond is conditioned. Stressed parents create stressed children, just as children of resilient parents tend to be more resilient themselves. Changes to the hypothalamus-pituitary-adrenal network can even change DNA and the function of genes, which makes the effects of stress long-lasting, even hereditary. It felt important to interrupt the cycle of a conditioned stress response. In an effort to promote resiliency, and peace, within our family, I turned to Dr. Dan for help.

The spotlight shifted back to Brennan. Dr. Dan didn't ask about the leukemia or cancer treatment, which surprised me. He asked about Brennan's friends and what things he liked to do.

While they were talking, I tried to remember what had worked to calm him in the past. All I could think of was what hadn't worked.

As an infant, he would squirm when coddled and scream harder when swaddled. Most kids calmed down in the car; he cried. I finally took him to the doctor to see if he was motion sick or had inner ear problems, something a nursing colleague had suggested.

"He's fine," the doctor reassured me. "Just go short distances at first."

"But I can't even get out of the driveway!" I said.

I finally concluded that Brennan detested being restrained. It might have been his craving for independence that got him upright and walking at nine months. When he was ten months old, we bought a light umbrella stroller for a trip to Seattle, where I was giving a talk. We buckled him in as we headed down the hill to the wharf. Within half a block, he screamed, arched his back, extended his long legs, hopped to his feet, and proceeded to walk down the hill, carrying the stroller on his back, the four sets of wheels facing skyward, twirling with freedom.

Dr. Dan worked with Brennan's preferences. "Let's let you drive the car. Are you ready?"

"Yes!" Brennan said, instantly scooting his chair up to the computer.

"I'm attaching an electrode to your arm to measure your muscles," Dr. Dan said, glancing up at me.

My whole body nodded agreement, telling him that I was familiar with galvanic skin response, which measured electrical impulses in the skin.

"Relaxing your arm makes the car move," he told Brennan as he attached the wires to the machine and computer. "Just let your arm hang over the side of the chair. The more relaxed you are, the faster your car will go. Let's try the breathing first."

Dr. Dan walked Brennan through closing his eyes and breathing slowly and deeply, so that he could feel what it felt like to relax all of his muscles. We both knew that once he turned on the computer screen, Brennan would tense up in preparation for the fun stuff.

"Okay, that's good, Brennan," he said. "Now let's see what relaxing looks like in color." A spiral on the computer screen grew bigger and more colorful the more relaxed he became, and it shrank to a tiny ball when Brennan shifted or squirmed in his seat.

"Okay, let's hop in the car," Dr. Dan said.

He coached Brennan to slow his breathing and relax his muscles, which triggered the traffic signal to change from red to yellow to green. Only after the signal turned green would the car take off, and the light had to stay green to keep it moving.

It was harder than it looked from the sidelines. I could see Brennan's brow crease as he concentrated, first as he tried hard to figure out how to get the car to move and then as he worked to relax his arm long enough to keep the light green.

He beamed when the car finally accelerated. He was driving! But every time his face lit up, the car stalled. It was the opposite of what he expected; he had to be relaxed in order to move forward. He had to let go in order to control.

The challenge of learning a new—and fun—skill kept Brennan coming back for several sessions with Dr. Dan. He had to practice staying relaxed, in the moment, even when his actions created reactions. Of course, the goal was that he would eventually teach himself to relax without needing the visual feedback of the screen.

And he did. In fact, Brennan put his new skill to use during clinic appointments. I didn't coach him or even remind him. He just closed his eyes, rested his head on my shoulder, took two deep breaths, and then nodded when he was ready for Sara to inject the asparaginase deep into his thigh.

"Wow, where did you learn that?" Sara asked.

"From Tiger Woods." Brennan grinned. "It helps him hit the ball farther."

I leaned back and smiled. Brennan and I had talked about how Tiger's mom, a Buddhist, had taught him self-discipline skills to help him concentrate and keep his composure on the golf course.

"Are you going to use it for golf, too?" Sara asked seriously.

"I don't need it for golf!" Brennan said as he puffed out his chest. "I can hit the ball as far as Tiger does."

Later that summer, at age five, Brennan was on the driving range, practicing with the golf pro. He finished each stroke with his torso facing the pin, his hands rolled over the shaft, and his right toe pointed into the ground.

"Way to go, Tiger!" called out a grandfatherly-looking member as he walked by on his way to the first tee.

CHAPTER 13

Who Is This Child?

In the single picture that snaps that summer into focus, the boys straddle the outside rim of the drained bathtub, facing each other. Brennan's eyes peek out from his chubby, ruddy cheeks, puffy from the steroids. His five-year-old smile is more certain than Tyler's. Both boys have blue eyes and sandy blond, fly-away hair. Brennan's hair is just growing back, coming in new and baby fine and sticking up in every direction, while Tyler's mind-of-their-own curls cover his ears. Having just finished his bath, Brennan wears long pajamas, even though it is summer. Space ships soar across his chest and Buddha-like tummy, while polar bears ice skate up and down his legs. Tyler wears jeans, the only time in his life when he did, and a white short-sleeved T-shirt with a big red airplane insignia on the front. Anything that moved by mechanical energy fascinated him; every shirt in his drawer was imprinted with either a construction machine or a mode of transportation. The setting auburn sun glances sideways through the frosted bathroom window. The moment fades as quickly as the day, but the image binds me forever to the summer of 1997.

I barely recognized Brennan that summer. Even Tyler would look at this photograph a decade later and ask, "Who is that?"

It was impossible to anticipate what would come next, much less peer into the future of the two boys posed for the camera in that shot. Brennan was in the midst of his first of two courses of delayed intensification. We had been going to the clinic every Monday, Wednesday, and Friday for chemotherapy to be shot into his leg, injected into his spine, or infused into his blood through his central line port-a-cath. We were there for an hour, hours, or much of

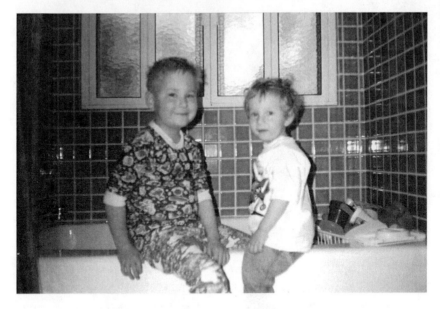

Brennan and Tyler, delayed intensification #1.

the day, as the infusions pumped drugs into his body to kill cancer cells and water to flush the chemicals from his kidneys. We read
books together, raced cars on the rug, drew pictures, played hang-
man, tic-tac-toe, and cribbage, and we watched an occasional *Tom
and Jerry* video.

We once watched *Charlie and the Chocolate Factory* on a long
day when he was in the hospital getting spinal chemotherapy.

"I don't want to watch this anymore," he said less than halfway
through the movie.

"Why not?" I asked.

"It's dumb."

I was surprised that he didn't say more, like offer an analysis of
what was lacking in the story. I suspect that the colorful costumes,
singing, and dancing were overstimulating his sensitive nervous system. The intrathecal chemotherapy often left him nauseous, lightheaded, and sensitive to light and sound. He would never watch the
movie again. I learned to not bring anything favorite to the hospital,
except for his blankie and buddy, which followed him everywhere,
for fear that the negative association would ruin it for him.

We were halfway through the DI#1, and we would soon be going to the clinic four days a week. We would go home and add more pills to his breakfast and bedtime snack and more snacks to his day. With extra weeks of prednisone and decadron, steroids particularly effective at killing fast growing lymphocytes, he would gain another six pounds during DI#2, an additional 10 percent increase of his body weight.

*   *   *

I don't know what compelled me to take the picture. It was just a normal day in the life of a family with cancer. The boys' faces are a little blurred in the photo, perhaps reflecting my own fatigue, my hurried nature, or my uncertainty of that time. I only took one picture. Normally, I would have taken several, to ensure that at least one came out after developing the 35 mm prints. In contrast, the bath toys piled into the rack spanning the tub appear crisp and colorful. On top of the pile is a yellow boat, a blue bucket with a red handle, and a plastic drinking cup with a red shovel sticking out. Buried underneath the pile was their favorite, the plastic yellow watering can that they regularly doused each other with. Fifteen years later, it would still be easier to see the toys than to look into their eyes.

I avoided this picture when the prints arrived in the mail. I flipped through them quickly, turning my head away from this single memory. It was hard to see Brennan bloated, gaining weight, and moon faced. Here was leukemia, ingrained in color on shiny paper. It could have been any child, like the picture of a little boy smiling from the page of one of the nursing or medical journals that arrived in my mail almost daily. But no, it wasn't a professional photograph, it was blurry. And it wasn't a poster child; it was my son. I flipped it over.

Whenever I see the picture, it brings back the heartache of that season, a time when I felt like I had no idea who this child, the one we were working so hard to save, was anymore. His identity seemed fuzzy. When I look into his blue eyes, searching for the little boy I know was buried somewhere amidst the daily rigor of treatment, meds, and routines, I try to glimpse life from his perspective—try to imagine what it was like for him growing up in a not-so-normal time of life.

*   *   *

These days, Brennan vacillated between extremes of frustrated, uncontrolled outbursts and can't-get-off-the-couch lethargy. The outbursts were intense but usually short-lived. When he had the energy, however, his verbal negotiations could relentlessly drag on for hours.

"We are done with this conversation, Brennan," I'd say.

"I know, but if you look at it my way—"

"It's going to stay the way it is."

"But—"

"Brennan, I can understand your frustration, but we are done talking about this."

"But you haven't even listened to me!" he'd wail. "You haven't heard the whole story!"

The anguish on his face would almost suck me back in.

I realized at the time that his outburst behavior and verbal manipulations reflected, in part, his need to control something, anything, in his new world. I watched how his nurse, Sara, offered him choices. She let him decide whether she should count to three before inserting the needle into his port or just put it in on the first count. He always chose the first count, the just-get-it-over-with option. Choices seemed to work better for her than they did for me.

Just two weeks after his diagnosis, he told me one evening as we lay together in his bed, "It is harder being on the receiving end than the giving end."

"What do you mean?" I asked, surprised that he could view his situation from anyone's perspective other than his own.

"I'm the one who has to get all the shots and things. I don't really have a choice."

It was one of the few times he verbally acknowledged the effort it took just to get through his days and the lack of control he felt. It was one of the few times that he spoke so clearly, or that I heard him so unmistakably, that I wrote it down in my journal.

Over time it would become easier to see the pattern of how Brennan's physical changes and aggression were expected side effects to the treatment. But at first, a part of me feared that this new experience was changing him in instinctive and elemental ways. Why couldn't I, Brennan's mother, find him inside of his own body? His behavior seemed such a metamorphosis from that first week, from the little yellow bird stuck inside of the house with no windows and no doors. I tried to give him credit; he had come a long way in adapting. But I was afraid my son would change forever and never return.

* * *

Memorial Day bloomed into a delightfully sunny day with temperatures in the mid-sixties, kicking my own determination into high gear. Duane and Brennan were watching a golf tournament on television.

"How about we go golfing instead of just watching golf?" I said. "It's a gorgeous day outside."

"I don't feel like it," Brennan replied.

"We could just play nine holes," I said, trying to tempt him.

"No."

"Well, how about miniature golf, then? We could go to Birdies, the place Laurie used to take you." Hearing no dissent, I said, "I will go look up the directions."

We always played mini-golf at the Mall of America or when we traveled. I had never been to a local outdoor course. But I was determined to get outside. It hadn't been this warm in eight months!

Brennan rarely turned down a golf outing. The summer he turned two, I videotaped him turning his back on the slides at the park to wander over and swing his dad's extra-long golf club. He gravitated toward any sport engaging hands to ball.

He went along with me that day, but he was distracted. We raced around the miniature golf course, skipping the setup and just hitting the ball to the hole and then quickly picking up and moving on to the next hole. I didn't even have time to write down the scores.

"I'm hungry," he announced as we sank the last ball into the eighteenth hole.

"How about we play one more round and then go get something to eat? Maybe I can beat you this time," I said, trying to appeal to his competitiveness. The day was too beautiful to go inside.

"No, I want to eat now," he replied, not even noticing the cloudless sky and first-of-the-season sun dancing through the trees and penetrating heat into his bare arms. We had driven thirty minutes only to race around the mini golf course in fifteen minutes.

We sat in a booth in a dark, deserted corner of the family-style restaurant next door for two hours. It was the middle of the afternoon; at least it didn't take long to get the food. Brennan ordered seconds and I watched him eat, smacking his lips as he shoveled in chips with melted cheese and then a cheeseburger and fries.

When Brennan was three years old, I took him to a faculty reception at the university. He was happy to come along and mingle with adults. He peered up over the white, cloth-draped table and observed the spread of deli meats and cheeses that lay neatly overlapping on silver serving platters. He turned to the dean's secretary and asked, "Do you have any aged cheddar cheese?"

So it surprised me when he begged us to buy Cheez Whiz that spring. I don't even know how he knew about the mainstay product of his father's childhood. There seemed to be no adequate substitute for the gooey, salty, processed cheese that stuck to the roof of your mouth but melted on everything else. "I have to have some NOW!" he would announce, standing solidly in place, flapping both arms down adamantly to his sides, his mouth puckered in place. "I *need* chips and melted cheese!"

He even smelled different now. Gone was the baby-soft hair and toddler-fresh smell. Maybe it's because he had so little hair to cling to the sweet-smelling Tom's baby shampoo. Or perhaps it's that the chemotherapy drugs were powerfully permeating each of his cells, like garlic does after an Italian dinner. Even the mosquitoes avoided him.

Brennan noticed it first. We were outside on the strip of grassy median in our neighborhood, playing baseball.

"Ouch!" I shrieked. "I'm getting eaten alive!"

"Keep moving," Duane said.

"Me too!" Tyler said, pointing to the big red welts already rising on his tender toddler arms.

"Not me!" Brennan commented matter-of-factly. And then he reflected, "I wonder why not?"

We stopped playing ball to analyze the situation. "If you are the only one they aren't biting, then maybe it's the chemotherapy," I said.

"Can they smell it?" Brennan asked.

No one knew the answer, but every time we played outside after that, the mosquitoes avoided Brennan, until he came off chemotherapy. He had a three-year mosquito grace period. Now that's a chemo perk in Minnesota!

On this day, post-mini golf, I stared across the table at Brennan as he ate. I missed the lively, talkative, dramatically expressive boy who seemed transformed overnight. It surprised me that I actually missed the challenge of keeping up with his constant questions and nonstop quizzes on every sports event and current player statistics.

"Who is the number one seeded player in the NFL this year?" he'd ask.

"I have no idea, Brennan!" I would reply, not even knowing what it meant to be "seeded."

"Take a guess," he would plead with me, wanting to banter or just to tell me I was wrong—again. And then, "Okay, fine. Who was the number one draft pick for the Diamondbacks this year?"

"Is that Arizona?"

"Yes, Mom," he would say with a sigh. "Now answer the question!"

I never got off easy.

Normally he would feel compelled to entertain me, a captive audience, at a lunch like this. Instead, he was silent. So I made desperate attempts to engage him in conversation, trying to keep the conversation on something other than treatment and illness.

"Do you know why we celebrate Memorial Day?" I asked.

"No, why?" he asked, his eyes focused on a chip.

I skimmed over an answer and then asked something more personally relevant: "Any thoughts on what you might want to do for your birthday in two weeks?"

"No."

I'd never imagined that I would lament the absence of his fiercely independent and tempestuous attitude. As I watched him, I pleaded with myself to find something, anything, in this boy that I recognized and loved. I doubt he saw my despair as I slouched in the oversized cushion and barely lifted my eyes to his. Chemotherapy was saving my son, but I felt I was losing him.

That's when I silently bargained with myself. Brennan had one more month of DI#1 and then two months of Interim Maintenance, a sort of respite, and then he would start kindergarten and DI#2 the same week in late August. I needed to have something to look forward to after we finished the first DI, or I wouldn't be able to face another repeat eight weeks later in the fall. I needed summer just as badly as he needed chips and cheese. Summer offered time for me to regroup after an intense year of teaching and meeting daily deadlines. And the flexible schedule provided me precious time to reconnect with the boys. Sure, I'd had lots of time with Brennan since his diagnosis five months earlier, but it was clinic time, hospital time, treatment time, and medication coercion and oversight time—not reconnecting time. I wanted to play, for his sake and mine. I wanted to be with him, not care for him. I wanted to be his mom, not his nurse.

Up until then, we had made no summer plans. My singular goal was to get through delayed intensification. I hadn't been able to look beyond tomorrow, although I knew what the road map laid out for us. Thirty more days suddenly seemed like a long time to have no goals other than "getting through." I decided, in the darkness of that maroon and mahogany space, that we needed to have something to look forward to. Even if we had to unexpectedly change our plans at the last minute, planning gave me hope.

"What do you think about going on a family vacation in July or August?" I blurted out.

"That's fine," Brennan said indifferently.

"Any place you would like to go?" I asked, searching my brain for possible locations that were kid-friendly, didn't require too much energy or too long of a drive or plane flight, and had available pediatric health care resources.

"I don't care," he said noncommittally.

I went home, called my sister-in-law, and that day booked airline tickets to Colorado. It felt safe to go to my younger brother's house, to be among family, to let the boys be kids and play with their cousins, and to have someone to share in the effort of just getting through the days. The grace of my sister-in-law rescued me from the pit of darkness. We came home with cowboy hats for the boys, which they wore for years. The memories cloak me in gratitude.

Deciding on a vacation was a turning point for me. Vacations were things that normal families did in the summer. I thought that if I could recreate a sense of normalcy and routine, the conditions in which Brennan felt comfortable and secure, I might rediscover my son.

CHAPTER 14

Finding Normal

As summer sauntered forward, Brennan lost interest in basketball, football, baseball, and golf. One afternoon he sat in the dark dining room, hunched over his notebook and markers. It was an unusual place for him to color, but he could see me outside with Tyler, and I could see him as two-year-old Tyler methodically filled and emptied his dump trucks in the flatbed of the truck-shaped sandbox, the late-afternoon sun streaming through his long golden curls. Gratefully, I breathed in the stillness and tranquility of my two boys as I soaked up the waning energy of the day's sun and planted my feet in the coolness of the earth. I felt grounded. It was summer, and it needed pacing, like the rhythm of a poem.

One early morning, Brennan handed me a thin strip of white paper, folded into a fan with precise creases.

"It's for you," he said.

He watched, leaning forward, as I unfolded it, one panel at a time. A vivid green flower, centered on the page, stood straight and tall on top of green grass and thick brown soil. I could almost smell its earthy fragrance. The flower's illuminated face shined through blue swirls and vertical streaks that filled the sky and completely surrounded it, with a splash of yellow sun shining down. The flower stood, centered and tall, like my son, flourishing in the midst of chaos, deriving nourishment from the sun and rain and earth. I imagined later that my careful unfolding of his picture gave new life to the strength that lay within. We both remained speechless as two tears slipped down my cheeks and I bent down to hug my son. "It's beautiful," I whispered in his ear. "I love you so much. I am so proud of you."

* * *

Brennan cel- ebrated his fifth birthday at the mid- point of DI#1. When Duane told me that he had to go on an out-of-town trip for work that week, I looked at him, incredulous. Had he forgotten the date?

"What could be more important than celebrating your son's life after cancer?" I asked.

I didn't get an answer. Either it was too late to change the commitment or the trip was more important. He didn't share how he felt about missing his son's birthday, per-

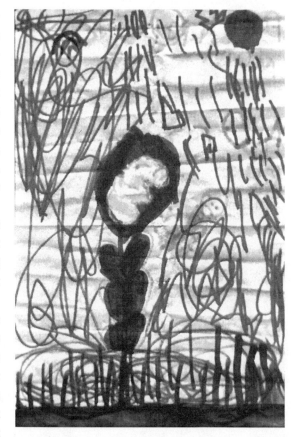

Brennan's flower, summer, Interim Maintenance.

haps because I wasn't very understanding of his dilemma. I doubt the lapse was intentional; birth dates just never quite registered with Duane as worth holding free. He would miss future birthdays, too, but this one seemed the most important to me.

Despite being in the midst of DI#1, or because of it, I wanted Brennan's birthday to be fun and frivolous and cancer-forgetting. Kit and Kaboodle, a guitar-playing duo who knew our boys from pre- vious gigs, sang "Grandma's Motorcycle Ride," "Hole in the Bottom of the Sea," and "Mittens Are So Spooky" outside on the patio for Brennan and fifteen friends and neighbors, all seated on chairs and laughing hysterically. Grandma and Grandpa drove the ninety miles to be there, and Laurie and Beth, our new nanny-to-be, came to help.

Brennan posed for a picture with Grandma and Grandpa with a big, laugh-out-loud smile, sitting at the kitchen table with his marble cake and melting raspberry chocolate chip ice cream, fuzzy sprouts of hair framing his round face.

And so it was that summer of 1997. We had fifty-six days of relative freedom, sandwiched in between DI#1 and DI#2. Brennan was still on daily treatment, but a less intense Interim Maintenance schedule meant appointments every two weeks instead of three to four times a week.

We filled our sandwich days with carefully selected excursions to the Turtle Derby races at the university, the Minnesota and Como Park zoos, and Pirate Ship and Triangle Park playgrounds.

"What do you want to do today?" I would ask in the morning after eyeing the weather report.

Most days we just did what we wanted to at the time. We walked down the street to the Walker Sculpture Garden and ran around the giant spoon and cherry sculpture and played hide and seek on the outdoor stage. We rode bikes and the tractor trike on the median, shot hoops on the patio, and built construction zones in the sandbox. During quieter times, I taught Brennan how to play cribbage and backgammon. He learned how to tally numbers in his head, and discovering the strategy of adult games at the age of five made him feel important. When he was tired, we read books together or he sat in the dining room or at his little table in the corner of the living room and drew pictures. I snapped a picture of Tyler napping in his crib with the book *What Do People Do All Day?* splayed open on his chest. Life began to feel normal. Smiles reemerged in photographs.

Choosing to do what we wanted, when we wanted, were the simple gifts of those eight weeks. I have pictures of me dressed for work, but I don't remember working. And my notes tell me we were in clinic six times in those eight weeks, but I don't remember being there. I don't even remember the meltdowns, though I'm sure there were some. The freedom and the fun times shared together imprinted themselves on my mind.

Without even realizing it, we had adapted. Ever since cancer had come home with us, I had carefully screened play dates and outside group activities. Brennan always came down with some virus shortly after climbing on community gyms and plunging through tunnels and bouncing balls at indoor play areas. Friends' kids had birthday parties at Chuck E. Cheese's, and I would ask, "Who is that?" We had our celebrations at home, playing Frisbee golf, hide and seek, and cops and robbers in the backyard woods.

* * *

As we usually did, I signed the boys up for swimming lessons at the outdoor pool at the golf club, timing the two weeks of lessons for when I expected Brennan would have more energy. Both boys loved the water, and we often stayed and swam afterward. Tyler fearlessly leapt off the low diving board into a floating "noodle" or receptive arms, while Brennan eyed the high dive.

"I'm going to do it today!" he announced one day.

"Great!" I said. "I'll stand right here and watch."

"Okay, see ya later!" he said more than once as he started to climb the ladder to the top. "Are you watching, Mom?"

"I'm watching! You're doing great, Brennan!"

He climbed up slowly—right hand, left foot, left hand, right foot—hands gripping the railing and feet securely planting themselves on each step before calculating the next move. Once at the top, he stopped and stretched his skinny arms out to each side rail, perched three feet high along the board. He inched forward, step by careful step, closer and closer to the bouncy end, the plank wiggling beneath his feet as he crept beyond the security of the rails.

I watched, careful not to talk or move, cautious to not distract him from his concentration. He stood perfectly still, toes lined up with the tip of the board, his arms stiffly extended down his sides. He stood there for a long time—a very long time. I waited.

He had seemed so confident when he started up. I imagined how high it must look to a five-year-old. I had once jumped from the high dive; he must have seen me do it, because I never went to the pool without the boys. Now it was his turn to feel the adrenaline pump his heart to the edge, launch his calves into a leap, and force the wind to squish his cheeks back to his ears. The anticipation of the impact with the water might cause him to wonder just how deep he would go and if he could hold his breath until he broke through the surface for that first gasping gulp of air.

I watched as he slowly, very slowly, backed up, inch by inch. He grabbed the rails and descended the steps, backing down, carefully planting his bare feet one methodical step at a time, until he reached the bottom. I waited for him to walk over to me.

"I can't do it today," he said, looking down at the dry, gray cement.

"Why not? You seemed so ready," I said as I wrapped the ocean blue beach towel with playful dolphins and sea turtles around his pale frame, now shivering from cold or fear. It was an overcast July day, and he had been in the water for more than an hour. My hand brushed his face gently to reassure him, and I felt the heat bursting from his skin. "Brennan, you are burning up! You have a fever! No wonder you don't feel up to jumping off a high dive!"

I helped him put on his T-shirt and called Tyler out of the pool. An hour later we were at the clinic with a temp of 103 degrees. Any fever over 101.5 degrees required that blood be drawn from his port-a-cath to culture for bacteria or fungal infection and a round of antibiotics.

We effortlessly reverted back to survival mode.

"I'm sorry you didn't get to jump today," I said once we were settled into the car on the way home.

"It's okay," Brennan said.

I sensed that his illness drove his apathy.

It would be weeks before he finally launched himself off that high dive. But he did it that summer, at five years of age, while on treatment for cancer. It was his goal, and he accomplished it. He had trusted his body to know when it was ready, and he had listened to it.

✳ ✳ ✳

That summer, Brennan also learned to ride a bike. At first the bike had training wheels, but he insisted they come off after the first week. The boys mostly rode on the sidewalk along the parkway. Brennan rode his bike and Tyler drove his tractor-trike, pulling a trailer filled with collected branches and pine cones. I was the bridge keeper, charging phantom quarter tolls, as they drove cross country, or at least to Wisconsin, where Grandma and Grandpa lived. I didn't think much of it until our new nanny, Beth, pointed out to me, a year later, that she had been surprised that we had given him a bike for his fifth birthday.

"Isn't that what five-year-olds do?" I said, clearly not getting her point.

"I was worried he would fall and hit his head or cut his leg," she said. She had worked with one of my graduate students in adult hematology/oncology and knew that patients with cancer risk bleeding and infection.

"But now I realize that you tried to keep his life as normal as possible," she said.

I nodded, surprised that she had thought about this. I tried to recall how seriously I had considered the risk. She was right. My mindset was programmed to normalcy that summer. Was I so intent on making life as normal as possible that I ignored the risk? Or was I finally letting go of the cautious nurse role and wrapping my arms around my son as his mother?

* * *

One Saturday that summer, Duane, Brennan, Tyler, and I decided to ride the Lake Harriett Street Car. Both boys loved trains and engines that blew whistles.

As we hopped aboard, the portly conductor called cheerfully out to Brennan, "Hey there, mate, gentlemen remove their caps when coming aboard."

Brennan, who was wearing a children's artist-designed cap with a visor, ignored him and sat down in the front seat that faced across the trolley so that he could see out the side window, right past the conductor.

The conductor turned in his seat and faced him. "I wear a cap because I'm the conductor," he said authoritatively, obviously bent on teaching this young man a lesson in etiquette. "And because I don't have much hair left." He laughed as he removed his shiny black conductor's cap to show us thinning gray hair. He brushed it aside and replaced his cap. "You are young enough not to need a cap."

The conductor sat facing Brennan and Duane, clearly enjoying his role. We were the first passengers on the trolley. Tyler and

I sat in the seat adjacent to Brennan and Duane, facing forward. I barely breathed. We waited in silence until Brennan, without a word, politely removed his cap and smiled broadly at the conductor.

Seeing Brennan's even balder head, with wisps of fuzz, the conductor sheepishly smiled and turned back to start the engine. "Well, then," he said, "let's get rolling!" He pulled the streetcar's whistle as the wheels slowly turned gear.

Brennan put his cap back on his head and, straight-faced, watched the houses and trees go slowly by outside the window.

I smiled inside at his new comfort level. Over time, baseball and football caps became his signature statement. He would leave twenty-six caps in his bedroom when he went off to college, and even now, as an adult, he resists taking them off when he enters public indoor spaces.

* * *

After treatment, Brennan mostly drew abstract designs, and he rarely talked about his thoughts or what it was like to have leukemia or to be on treatment. When I asked him about what he remembered or about his thoughts or feelings, he always mentioned the back medicine. Other than that, he said he didn't think about it anymore. "That was in the past," he would say.

Nine years after treatment ended, in a one-page paper in his high school English class, he wrote:

Little did he know he would never be a normal kid. When he was four, he was diagnosed with leukemia. He'll never be a normal kid, his parents thought. He'll never live a normal life, they thought. He might not make it through, they thought. The boy, on the other hand, thought, it's no big deal. I'll make it through. I'll live a normal life anyway. But no matter how hard he tried, he couldn't be like the other kids. While they were living their carefree childhood lives, he missed half a year of school and had to be monitored constantly. When he wasn't being monitored, he was doing his best to fit in with the other kids. He went to school, played sports, hung out with friends, but no matter how hard he tried to convince himself, he was not like the other kids. The one thing he was sure of, however, was that he would get through it. He fought hard for three long years.... After it was all over he finally took the opportunity to make up for lost time. He wanted to live a normal life, and now he finally could. He was right, it was no big deal, he made it through, and he lived a normal life. However, he still lives with the memory of those not so normal three long years of his young life.

Normal was an illusion driven by our expectations. We had to learn to expect the unexpected, adjust to uncertainty, adapt to abrupt changes in plans, and accommodate disruption. While it seemed chaotic at the time, we learned to live in the moment, not knowing what the next moment might bring, and to breathe through the challenges, because sometimes that was all we could do.

When our frantic pace calmed a bit that summer, I had time to stop and look around, to see where we were headed, and even to reflect on where we had been. It was like resurfacing after a high dive jump. I took stock of where I was and then got out of the way.

The road map still directed our daily routine, but how we lived was up to us. Cancer was only part of our identity; it may be shaping us, but it couldn't define us. We were a family living with cancer, not just a cancer family surviving treatment.

CHAPTER 15

Sailing Forward

Just before kindergarten started, Brennan drew a bright red sun, glowing against the deep blue sky, hovering just above the green horizon, a yellow shadow marking its ascent.

I, too, looked forward to resuming a routine, getting through his second delayed intensification and coming to the end of the eleven-month aggressive treatment phase. In November, Brennan would start twenty-eight months of a less intense and more routine maintenance phase. Long-term maintenance, here we come!

But first we had to get there.

Kindergarten and DI#2 started the same week. Brennan's classmates went full-day, but we negotiated for half-day so that he could be at the clinic for treatment three afternoons a week. The other two days he rested at home.

On the day of his first afterschool clinic appointment, I arrived early to pick him up from school. I was surprised to find the classroom empty. And then I heard dozens of high-pitched, energetic voices shouting to each other outside. A back door to the kindergarten room exited two steps down to the playground. A posse of flushed faces and waving arms sped past the big picture windows of the bright and sunny kindergarten room. I could almost feel the late–August wind whipping through their sweaty hair.

I turned back, smiling contentedly, inhaling the stillness and silence of the long rectangular room, carved on one end with a cooking nook and a reading loft. A visual graph of construction paper ice cream cones caught my eye. Twelve scoops of chocolate ice cream piled high on one cone, clearly winning as the favorite flavor the kids had chosen the day before on their field trip. I imagined all twenty

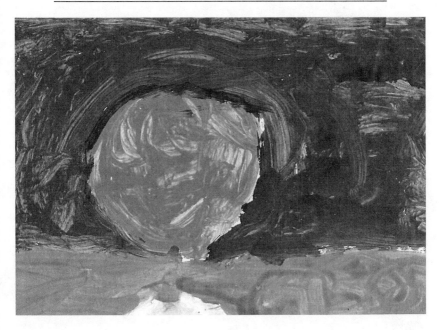

Brennan's red sun rising.

kids sitting around the ice cream shop's outside tables, mouths wide open, licking the creamy treat, drips rolling down their chins in the warm summer breeze. Brennan couldn't have dairy at night, so I was happy he could enjoy this treat with his class.

I looked up and saw, stretching from corner to corner above the windows, a rainbow of colors and jumbo-size letters and numbers, all pledging academic success. It suddenly dawned on me, standing alone in the center of the classroom, that this school was preparing these children for a secure future, for a life beyond kindergarten. They expected these children to move on, to learn and grow—and live. The realization snatched my breath. I had been so focused on just getting here—to this school, to this day, and to the next treatment. I was literally living from one moment to the next; the future was out there somewhere, beyond any horizon I could see.

I turned to watch the kids outside running off their infectious energy. Brennan was among them. I whispered aloud, pleading to God, to my guides in the universe, to the oncology team, to the faculty of the school, to whomever would hear me: "Please see him through to graduation."

For just a brief flash, I imagined Brennan standing on stage to receive his diploma. It seemed such a finite wish. Something concrete, measurable, and expected, like the findings from my research, carefully calculated from and confirmed by stacks of data and stories collected over years. I instantly believed in my son's future. The vision wasn't of a bald-headed child with cancer. It was of a child with potential, just like the other nineteen children in his kindergarten class. He would need goals and direction, a plan. I felt an intense purpose. I wanted him to learn, to have motivation to learn, and to enjoy learning. I wanted him to have friends, to fight over playground equipment, to learn teamwork, to find his strengths, and to rise to his challenges.

My heart swelled into my throat as the kids suddenly burst through the back classroom door, laughing and calling out to one another as they lined up to wash their hands in the classroom sink, ready for lunch. Brennan would be the only one leaving for the afternoon. We were both okay with that.

*   *   *

I suppose it was unrealistic to expect that we would get through DI#2 without an acute exacerbation of *something*. After all, we were exposing his body to intense, immune-suppressing, grenade-launching chemotherapy and to novel and virulent germs harbored by little hands clutching group-shared pencils, crayons, books, and door handles.

Over the course of treatment, many people would ask me, "Why don't you home school him?"

I usually just stared at them, at a loss for words. I should have retorted, "Can you imagine what it would be like to tutor Mussolini or Napoleon Bonaparte?" I could easily predict who would win each day's debate about any proposed lesson plan or agenda. In fact, we would probably spend the entire day debating why we even needed an agenda. "No way!" I would eventually reply to the home school questioners, softening the intensity of my response with a lame "I have my own career, thankfully."

We paid the price in germs.

After a month of school, Brennan woke up one morning with

severe hip pain and a bronchitis that required inhaled nebulizer treatments.

"We have the nebs covered," I said to the oncologist. "We'll just take turns."

Tyler had started on nebs four times a day that summer after a torrential rainstorm blew out a five-foot window in our basement and flooded it with a half-foot of water. The mold counts in our house skyrocketed to 400,000 per cubic millimeter, despite prompt wet vacuuming and clean-up efforts, and I discovered that the boys, like me, were very allergic to mold.

I had no clues about what was causing Brennan's hip pain. I watched him recline on the white paper–clad examining table, propped up on an elbow, just as he had on the day of diagnosis eight months earlier. Although I considered it, I knew that a recurrence of leukemia was unlikely during such an intense treatment phase.

The oncologist ordered a CT scan to rule out avascular necrosis. Thankfully, Brennan didn't have that but a more resolvable toxic synovitis or inflammation of the joint itself. We just had to wait for it to improve. Although he was disappointed to miss six days of school, he was in too much pain to walk. With rest, antibiotics, and anti-inflammatory meds, both his bronchitis and hip pain resolved within two weeks.

Other than the eerie similarity to the leg pain at diagnosis, I wasn't particularly worried about this setback. It helped that the symptoms didn't drag on without an explanation, although for Brennan the pain was probably more distressing than the cause. The prompt scans and the oncologist's optimism reassured me. I reminded myself that he would get another bone marrow biopsy in just a few weeks, and we would know for sure about any potential for relapse. I was learning to live with uncertainty and to expect the unexpected. This was just another storm, par for the course of treatment.

As he rested at home, Brennan drew a second sailboat, colored in bold reds and dark blues, sailing at a 45-degree angle, as if trying to stay afloat. Next to it, lightning bolts zapped horizontally through black-tinged storm clouds, and red and blue rain, like exclamation points, descended vertically in torrents. Surrounding the sails were two red and royal blue auras, perhaps providing protection from the storms. A bright yellow sun peeked through at the bottom as if it were an afterthought or perhaps an expectation. Underneath the boat, in black marker, Brennan had written "MOM" and "BRENNAN."

I was thankful that he knew I was there for him.

* * *

Tyler started preschool three weeks after Brennan started kindergarten. He was only two and a half years

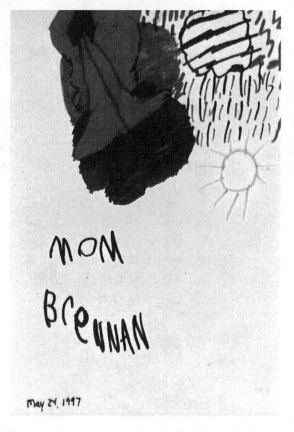

Brennan's sailboat sailing through storms and sun.

old, but we thought it would be good for him to have new experiences and new playmates of his own and his own routine. He seemed excited and ready, dressed in a smile and a favorite button-down striped shirt, a decorated ice cream bucket dangling from his hand.

The phone calls started sometime after the first few weeks of school, after the onset of Brennan's hip pain.

"Tyler seems distressed when we have to do anything outside of the classroom," the experienced teacher said. "He cries when we leave the room to go to some other activity."

The two teachers had tried preparing him for what would come next, taking his hand and walking with him, and even having him lead the class, but nothing seemed to work.

"Maybe if you come and sit in the classroom in the rocking chair while he is here, your presence will calm him," she suggested.

I agreed to try, and I spent four Fridays in the classroom, watching Tyler, reading on my own, trying to be unobtrusive but present. He walked over to me on occasion, seeking reassurance, but otherwise he played quietly on his own or with the other children. I don't remember him crying.

The teacher called back a week or two later. She seemed apologetic, as if she was responsible for him not adjusting better. "Maybe it's too early to start him in preschool. Maybe there is just too much going on in his life right now." She quickly added, "Although we could keep trying."

"I appreciate your efforts," I said. "But I agree; he may not be ready. He's had a lot of uncertainty and stress, both with his brother's treatment and his own health issues this summer. Maybe we are expecting too much of him." Tyler was still getting used to the invasiveness of nebulized facemask treatments four times a day and taking new medications, including prednisone, for his reactive airway disease. "I have no problem with taking him out of school right now. It's okay. We'll try again next year."

I breathed a sigh of relief as I hung up the phone. The teacher seemed relieved, too.

Tyler had always been sensitive. One day that fall, after I enforced a time-out for Brennan, Tyler sat on his scooter looking sad and pouty. After a few moments, I walked over to him, bent down, and gave him a hug.

"How's Tyler feeling?" I asked.

He silently looked down at his stationary feet.

"What's Tyler thinking?"

He didn't move.

"Hmm. It must be hard for Tyler to see Brennan get scolded." I wasn't sure I was right—it could be that he was just sad that he'd lost his playmate of the moment. But when he let out a sob and jumped into my arms, I knew he was relieved that I understood.

"It's okay to feel sad, but Brennan will be all right. And you aren't the one in time out!"

With that, he laughed and climbed out of my arms to resume his scooter ride, by himself.

A few weeks later, he started trembling in my arms after getting a flu shot. Instead of crying, like most two-year-olds would, his little body just vibrated. I noted in my journal how the patterns to suppress emotions and withdraw start so early.

Studies show that siblings often have a harder time adjusting than the child with cancer. Older siblings typically do better because they can appreciate the positive effects, such as closeness and compassion. Brennan did get more attention that year, but I tried hard to give both boys alone time with Mom. If anything, I became even more protective of Tyler, as he was often the convenient target for Brennan's aggression.

From a very young age, Tyler showed remarkable empathy toward others and animals. Although I will never know how his brother's leukemia shaped him, he was acutely aware of the change in his routine and in our new family dynamic. He might have needed the comfort and safety of home that year.

Years later, he would transfer colleges in his second year to commute from home, leaving behind his first dorm experience for the comfort of sleeping in his own bed at night. Perhaps venturing forth on his own terms is simply more in keeping with his disposition. I'm just glad that we could allow him to experience life at his own pace.

* * *

I learned that fall that there would always be storms. Cancer generated some. Life added others.

Just about the time Brennan started feeling better, I noticed that our tabby cat, Churchill, spent most of the day curled up in the corner of my tiny, overstuffed closet. I found him one day nestled on top of a pile of shoes blanketed by a forgotten pink nightgown that had fallen off its hook. Dark gray cat hair covered his warm and cozy nest. "How long have you been escaping here?" I asked him, a hint of worry and guilt in my tone. "We miss you." I gently picked him up and cradled his toasty body, his fur frizzed with static. "Is life really this stressful for you now? Have I neglected you?" I gave him a little extra love and attention that day.

The next day he quietly appeared in the kitchen for breakfast, but as he approached his dish, he coughed. It was a pathetically weak and raspy cough for such a sturdy tomboy in the prime of his life. Startled, I gingerly picked him up. I could feel his prominent ribs. And this time I couldn't toss it off to a growth spurt, as I had with Brennan.

"Our dog had a cough like that. He had bronchitis," Beth said, as we all stood in the kitchen blankly staring at the cat. I nodded, grabbing on to that hope, and vowed to call the vet once his office opened.

It was Halloween, and a Friday. Brennan and I set off for school, stuffing his green felt-covered foam golf course costume into the back seat. I snuck in a few hours of work in between the school parade and assembly and his afternoon chemotherapy infusion. As soon as he was disconnected from his infusion, I packed up, anxious to leave, when he reminded me, "But Mom, we have to play a game!"

"Brennan, I'm sorry, but I have to get Churchill to the vet *today* before they close. There isn't time to play basketball." He looked sullen and dejected. Feeling guilty for cutting out the only reward of his multiple weekly treatments, I caved in. "Oh, okay, a short game— 25 points wins!" He hesitated, until I reminded him that we had trick-or-treating too that night.

He always knew when I "let him win." But my heart wasn't into the competition that day. I couldn't let Churchill suffer until Monday, and I couldn't wait that long to find out what was wrong. As we pulled into the driveway, I quickly exchanged the kid for the cat and raced off to the next stop of the day.

"It doesn't look good," the vet said. "The x-ray shows a total white out of both of his lungs. I can draw off some of the fluid with a needle. It goes in between his ribs, into the pleural space just outside of his lungs." I listened intently, while he continued. "The fluid probably will come back. We can send the sample out for diagnostics to see if it is infection or something else."

Something else. How many times had I heard that phrase before in my work? I hesitated, wondering how long I could let this go on. *But I'm not ready yet; I'm not ready to let him go.* It was all too sudden. And he was only thirteen; our other cat had lived to be fifteen. Churchill was so much more vibrant and healthy. I nodded and agreed to "the tap," which would become a weekly and then biweekly event. I arranged Churchill's lung taps in between Brennan's spinal taps for his chemotherapy. The pathology report had come back with mesothelioma cells. Churchill and his cancer needed me, too.

It wasn't until Brennan finished DI#2 and started long-term maintenance, and until the Christmas season was over and quarter grades were in, that I could come to grips with saying good-bye to Churchill. It helped to have time to grieve before having to say a final good-bye. I had to let him go and relieve him of the repetitive and painful treatments. I couldn't make him hang on any longer just for me. I didn't even consider chemotherapy. I had allowed myself, and the boys, time to say good-bye, and now it was time to let go.

Somehow, in the midst of Brennan's illness, Tyler's stress at pre−K, and the cat's impending demise, I managed to submit a research grant with a new team, teach two classes, and graduate two master's students. The day before Thanksgiving, after I dropped Brennan off at school, I stopped by Starbucks to read a student's thesis before heading to work. As I got up to leave, I set my wallet on top of the stack of papers on the table and reached over the back of the chair to pick up my scarf and put on my coat. In those split seconds, a stocky, dark-skinned man in a black, down coat slipped through the door, grabbed my wallet, and bolted back out. I yelled, "STOP!" as I grabbed for his coat and tore off the hood. Then I ran out the door after him, hood in hand, and managed to get the license plate number of the black sedan waiting for him at the corner before it took off.

The thief ditched the stolen car within an hour but was caught two weeks later as he tried to cash my check at the bank using my driver's license. Instead of going to work that day, I headed home to call the banks and credit card companies and order a new driver's license. As I walked in the door, Brennan jumped up from the kitchen table, ran up to me, and handed me a one-dollar bill.

"Here, Mom," he said. "It's all I have, but you can have it."

I still have that dollar bill tucked away. It meant millions to me.

In the scheme of things, losing a wallet was minor. It was just another blip. It was the following week, in the deep December Minnesota cold, when I lost my earmuffs, that I cried.

✽　✽　✽

When we finally reached long-term maintenance, it felt anti-climactic. We didn't celebrate; it wasn't like Brennan was coming off treatment, just that the intensity and frequency of clinic visits and chemotherapy infusions would become more routine, standardized over three-month cycles. For the next twenty-eight months, Brennan would be on the same three-month cycle of daily and weekly oral chemotherapy, monthly prednisone and intravenous vincristine pulses, plus the triple intrathecal chemotherapy once every three months. Instead of weekly back medicine injections, we would go four times *a year.* All eighty-four days now descended on a single road map page. His bone marrow was clear. Relief was reward enough.

And Brennan loved school. In his semester report, the teachers commented on his happy morning smile, positive attitude, confidence, independence, eagerness to learn, and even inner strength and calmness, an ability to take things in stride. I don't know how he did it. I wished I had his strength, resilience, and perspective. He thrived at school because his teachers offered him freedom within structure, clear expectations with certain outcomes, and a sense of security—certainty that didn't exist in the world of cancer treatment.

As we ended the first year of treatment, Brennan drew his third sailboat. With a bright blue sail and bold red hull, it was centered and upright on calm, royal blue water. It sailed directly toward a lively red lighthouse that beckoned with yellow swirls of light. On the other side of the lighthouse was white, open space, emptiness, an unknown journey ahead.

For the first time all year, I sat in the living room with Brennan's folder of pictures. I stared, aching, at the little yellow bird, crouching alone in the rafters of the house. I smiled at the toys and colorful lights outside, grateful for the windows and doors. In two days, he had redesigned his house.

I reflected on how my son found strength in his drawings, in his ability to find light in the darkest of days. I marveled at his flower, rising from the earth in the midst of chaos, straight and secure.

His sailboats appeared as we gained distance, each one working hard to stay afloat. Storms had been our teachers. We had learned to catch the wind in the sail and tack right through them, gaining momentum on our journey.

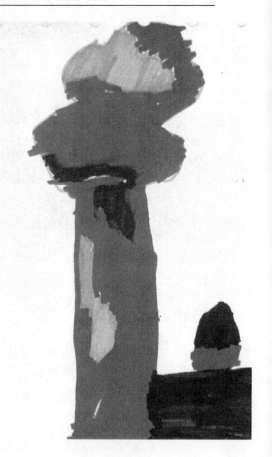

Brennan's lighthouse to guide his sailboat.

PART II

Treatment Years 2–3
The New Normal

The oak fought the wind and was broken,
the willow bent when it must and survived.
—Robert Jordan, *The Fires of Heaven*

Chapter 16

Expectations

When we were young, my sister and I constructed leaf houses in the front yard. Our commissary was the pile of crisp, fallen maple and elm leaves of sullen browns and playful reds and yellows that our father vigorously raked in a mound for us. We dug out our coats and hats from the deep recesses of the hall closet, and as the brisk winds swirled, we corralled the leaves to shape the foundation and rooms. We lovingly designed our houses, season after season, enacting our dreams with innocent and invincible expectations. We focused on the moment, bringing joy to our play.

Being young and naïve, we didn't anticipate the storms, and inevitably we would wake up to scattered leaves and loss. Sometimes we chose to rebuild our leaf house; other times we simply moved on and let go of our dreams. We were practicing for our future, even though we couldn't yet conceptualize the fragility of life.

* * *

Just before Christmas, the oncology clinic hosted a private event at Dayton's department store annual holiday display so that kids with cancer could greet the Nutcracker characters and Santa without getting exposed to the typical winter germ pool. We were surprised to run into friends we had known in Chicago nine years earlier. Their daughter had had leukemia then, at age two.

"Hey, what are you guys doing here?" Duane and I asked hesitantly.

"Caelhan relapsed again," both parents replied, matter-of-factly, as if they weren't sure how we would take the news. Caelhan, the older and more experienced cancer survivor, introduced herself to

Brennan, and they retreated to the bench against the wall to sit down and talk while her mom explained the situation to us.

"She relapsed when she was eight, four and a half years off treatment, and now again, at eleven. She's scheduled for a bone marrow transplant in January."

I tried to be encouraging, but all I could think was, *When can we ever feel safe?*

* * *

The holiday season was far more joyous than it had been the previous year, when Brennan was sick and we didn't know why, and my father's cardiac recovery was uncertain. One year later, Brennan was alive and moving on with his childhood, and my father was alive and adapting to his new physical limitations. They both looked more like themselves: both had slimmer physiques and more energy. Brennan's hair was growing back, too—thin, but now a half-inch long.

No one talked about the previous Christmas, when Brennan had spent an entire day huddled in the dark hotel room, wrestling with stomach pain and exhaustion, and then insisting after dinner that we go ice skating with his new skates.

Instead of skating this Christmas, we stayed inside and played Schmier, our family's traditional German card game. Laughter leapfrogged around the table as bidding wars ensued. The sharp contrast from one year to the next, from age four to five, from heartbreak to joy, gave me hope.

* * *

After the holidays, as Caelhan's family began their month-long hospital stay, we hopped a plane to a family wedding in eastern Wisconsin. We left on January 9, the one-year anniversary of Brennan's diagnosis.

The night before the wedding, we met college friends for dinner. Brennan ate very little and then lay down across three chairs at the restaurant while the adults talked. When he did the same thing the next day at the wedding reception, I stroked his back as we chatted with the bride's father, thinking that he was tired or bored. But on the one-hour plane trip home, he lay across my lap and vomited into the paper air sickness bag.

I assumed it was motion sickness, a phenomenon that had started with intrathecal treatment, but it didn't get better once we landed. I put him to bed when we got home and let him skip school on Monday, thinking he might have a virus.

He wasn't any better on Tuesday, so I skipped my class prep and took him in to the clinic. His hemoglobin had dropped from his normal of 12.5 to 9.0 g/dl in ten days. Even more striking was his lowered platelet count of 77,000 μL. His astute oncologist held his chemo, including his oral meds, and drew blood to test for sepsis, mononucleosis, Epstein Barr Virus, cytomegalovirus, and parvovirus. Everything was negative.

"Come back in on Friday," Dr. Steve advised, which gave me three days to stew over the symptoms. I taught class on Wednesday but stayed home on Thursday. Brennan's behavior had changed and he had become lethargic. I worried.

On Wednesday I confided to my research assistant, also a nurse, "He barely moves. He even plays cribbage lying down because he doesn't have the energy to sit up."

Lynne patiently listened as I processed out loud.

"And he's stopped talking! It's so unlike him."

Lynne's daughter was one of our fill-in sitters. She knew his silence was significant.

"His somnolence worries me the most. Maybe it's hepatitis or something neurological." I hesitated to conjecture, but Lynne would understand my compulsion to analyze and my need for a sounding board.

"Yes, it could be either," she agreed, her voice soft.

I felt a little less neurotic.

On Friday, Dr. Steve did an abdominal ultrasound. Brennan's two-pound weight gain and expanding tummy from abdominal fluid retention wasn't as obvious to me as it was to his doctor. How could I see subtle change while I hovered over my son hour by hour?

"He has veno-occlusive disease [VOD] of his liver," Dr. Steve announced with just a hint of excitement in his voice as he maneuvered the ultrasound over Brennan's right side, just below his ribcage.

He paused and stepped back. "We recently received a memo about the risk of VOD with kids on 6-TG. Brennan is the fifth child on this protocol to get VOD, all at about the one-year anniversary."

At that point I didn't soak up the potential risk of this finding. My mind busily occupied itself contemplating 6-TG as the cause and being thankful that he had stopped chemo on Tuesday. Brennan's hemoglobin had fallen even farther, to 7.4 g/dL. I appreciated that Dr. Steve had trusted his instinct when the evidence hadn't been conclusive three days earlier.

"So, what's next?" I asked after he explained the physiology of how some of the small veins get obstructed and reverse their blood flow, causing the liver to enlarge.

"We will hold his chemo until his hemoglobin and platelets go back to normal and we'll watch his liver enzymes. They can take longer to come back down. Then he will switch to 6-MP, the standard thiopurine." Because of the experience of the first four children, he explained, the leukemia protocol had been revised to reduce the dosages of 6-TG and to switch to 6-MP if liver abnormalities occurred. The clinical trial network fostered quick communication and prompt action, although reducing dosages in the clinical trial ultimately didn't prevent the incidence of VOD.

Brennan was one of the lucky ones. He didn't require hospitalization or transfusions. Of the 206 children participating in the study who eventually developed VOD (20 percent of the kids on 6-TG, despite dose reductions), three went into acute liver failure. Although no one died, one child required a liver transplant and one was hospitalized in the intensive care unit for three weeks.

After two weeks of his chemotherapy being postponed, Brennan's hemoglobin and platelets were back to normal, although his liver enzymes fluctuated up and down throughout the remaining two years of treatment. I don't know if there are long-term consequences. I warned him when he came off treatment about the risks of drinking alcohol and the effects drugs could have on his liver.

"But I'm only eight!" he replied.

* * *

Brennan went back to school after three full weeks at home. The picture of him standing in front of his science fair project reveals a pale, skinny boy who's smiling because he was told to. His white uniform shirt hangs crookedly over his taut, distended tummy. He slouches at a slant, his head tilted and his left hand tucked up into his long sleeve, as if he barely has enough energy to remain upright. But he was getting better.

The untimely VOD dredged up the uncertainty and vulnerability of the previous year. Fears of losing my son hurtled back to the surface, reminding me not to assume that life was anywhere near "normal." Hypervigilance triumphed once again.

Within a week of going back to school, back on full-dose chemotherapy, Brennan woke up with shaking chills and a 105-degree fever. I was scheduled to give a talk that day at noon for the cancer center, but by then, he was being admitted to Children's Hospital. His white blood cell count was quickly rising, with 98 percent neutrophils, strongly suggestive of sepsis, a systemic bacterial infection.

"Don't leave me, Mom!" he said, tears streaming down his cheeks. It was one of the few times I saw him cry throughout treatment. He shivered under the sheets in the hospital bed and huddled closer to me.

"I am right here," I said, lying next to him, holding him. "I won't leave." I was so relieved that he could tell me that he was afraid.

It was only his second hospitalization, but I knew the routine: triple intravenous antibiotics, close observation of circulatory and organ failure from septic shock, and the wait for blood culture results. It took twenty-four hours to stabilize his diastolic blood pressure, which had dropped to thirty when it should have been at least sixty. I stayed with him, reassured him, and explained what to expect. Duane assumed nighttime duty.

Brennan started to feel better after forty-eight hours of antibiotics and intravenous fluids. When Laurie came to visit, I slipped out and wandered down the hall to sit and deliberate with one of the oncologists about how to discriminate between bacterial and viral infections. It was more of an academic question; I was hoping to learn something. All infections were risky for cancer patients, but bacterial infections always required hospitalization and intravenous antibiotics, whereas viral infections could be treated at home by managing symptoms and monitoring for secondary bacterial infections.

"If the blood cultures come back negative, does that mean this is viral?" I asked. "Everything else seems to suggest bacterial infection."

"We have to treat it as if it could be bacterial," she said.

That made clinical sense, I agreed. I was thankful for their prompt action, and I was relieved that I wasn't trying to solve this alone at home.

Just a few hours later, when I went home for lunch and to check in with Tyler and Beth, fatigue and chills suddenly overwhelmed me. I called the oncologist before crawling into bed. "I think we have our answer. I seem to have what Brennan has. And Tyler isn't feeling well, either."

They sent Brennan home that afternoon. It could have been both bacterial and viral, but influenza peaked that February, and they didn't want us contaminating the rest of the kids on the oncology floor.

I stayed in bed, miserably ill, for three days, unable to care for the boys. Having a nanny was a lifesaver. Tyler ended up in the emergency room, back on prednisone for his asthma, and it took all three of us weeks to fully recover.

In the first three months of long-term maintenance, Brennan had already had two significant illnesses and six weeks of chemotherapy held. And this was the less aggressive treatment phase.

Over the next two years of treatment, he would have ten more documented illnesses, including three out-of-town emergency room visits for fevers, parvovirus (Fifth's disease), direct exposure to chicken pox (which causes severe risk in ALL), and four more holds or dose modifications of his chemotherapy. The more holds on chemotherapy, the greater the risk of relapse. But dying from complications of treatment, usually infection, was just as great a risk as dying from the leukemia.

Sometime that January, in between crises, I met Caelhan's mom on the bone marrow transplant unit. They were about two weeks past the transplant infusion (in which stem cells donated from her younger sister were infused), and Caelhan was having severe mouth pain, nausea, diarrhea, and fatigue from the sloughing of her gastrointestinal tract, an expected but miserable effect of transplant. She slept, with the help of morphine, while her mom and I quietly talked, sitting side by side on a bench in the hallway, close enough to hear if she called out.

"How are you doing?" I asked, leaning closer, intent on knowing what it was like for my friend.

"It's hard to see her sick, but we're managing," she said. As her fingers fiddled with each other in her lap, she filled me in on the details of the symptoms they were dealing with and how Caelhan's counts were responding. I noted all the facts, filing them away in my mind.

And then Carol abruptly and passionately started talking about her daughter's first treatment. "I worried about relapse when she came off treatment," she said, as if anticipating that someday I would, too.

I listened attentively, ignoring the midday hustle of phones ringing and staff scurrying about delivering meds and IVs and responding to call lights.

"I kept thinking, *What if?*" She looked up at me and I nodded in understanding. "As time went on, it got better. When she did relapse, four years later, I realized how much precious time I had wasted in worrying. We could have been playing and enjoying life!" Her eyebrows rose and her petite spine straightened, as if she was just realizing it again for the first time. I kept silent.

"In no way did it prepare me for the event," she said strongly and convincingly. "I have since learned to live each day with joy, thankful for the moments we have, joyful for the times we share." She paused and quietly reflected, her eyes softening. "After the second treatment, life was much more fun. There really was joy. And even now, with her second relapse and bone marrow transplant, we can still appreciate the good days. I learned that."

I soaked up the flood of her emotions. Then I walked quickly back to my office to write down what she had said. This new perspective jolted me awake. I've always been an optimist, but joy had seemed a liberal emotion since Brennan's diagnosis. It wasn't that I was unhappy. I just had an intense focus on what needed to get done.

I had always been a happy and outgoing child, and I loved sponta-neous playtime and meaningful moments with my children. My con-versation with Caelhan's mom reminded me that sharing smiles and laughter and moments were more important than all of the doing that cancer demanded.

"Work now, play later" had been my mantra all my life. The prob-lem with that training was that "later" rarely came once Duane and I filled our lives with responsibilities and to-do lists that never seemed to get checked off. So I added "happy times" to my list. I had to make room for joy.

And then I tried to let go of my own expectations. Because hap-piness comes when we let go, not when we try to control.

Which, of course, never completely happened. An analytical mind wants to order things, make sense of things, make the unknown known. But after meeting Carol that day, I tried harder to let go of the outcome and my expectations for a particular outcome. I focused on feeling joy in the moment, bookended by plans.

CHAPTER 17

Always on Call

"Where are you going on spring break?" another mother asked me as our boys peeled off coats, hats, boots, and mittens in the cramped coat room before class.

"To work!" I replied as optimistically as I could get myself to feel. I hadn't even thought of going anywhere else. Brennan finally felt well, and I was preoccupied with finishing the academic quarter, getting winter quarter grades in, and completing a talk and a paper for a national award I was receiving in May. I had been at my office all day every Saturday since New Year's Day. And besides, faculty didn't get spring break.

"Is everyone else going out of town?" I asked, suddenly aware of the escalating hubbub of flight, skiing, and beach itineraries. Would the boys feel let down if we didn't go anywhere? I was tired, and I felt ready to move on with my own career after fifteen months of merely surviving. My mind froze the chatter and blew it away with a sigh.

* * *

Not traveling turned out to be a blessing. Brennan spent the two weeks leisurely playing at home with Beth and Tyler while I caught up at work. The following week, my father was hospitalized for emergency bowel surgery. I didn't hesitate. With my talk just a month away, I tossed pictures and slides in the backseat of my car and drove the four hours to be with my parents.

"I can't believe you brought work!" my sister said. I couldn't tell if she was being critical or just more realistic. After all, I had learned to pluck time from every open window to do what needed to be done.

The surgery went smoothly, but abdominal incisions involve a long recovery, and we worried about the effects of anesthesia on my father's heart, permanently weakened from his heart attack eighteen months earlier. Even more unnerving, the pre-op chest x-ray had found an ominous spot on his lung. I never did get to work on my talk; instead, my three siblings and I all swooped in to support Mom and help Dad manage his abdominal pain and regain his strength by walking the halls.

After the initial crisis was over and Dad was recovering, we went home, leaving Mom in the hotel and responsible for keeping us informed. A couple of weeks later, knowing they would be there alone for Easter, longer than they had expected to stay, Duane and I decided to surprise them with a weekend visit. As Duane loaded up the car with the boys and overnight gear, I sneakily hid some plastic Easter eggs with coins and candy and locked up the house.

We stopped at my parents' house, which was halfway in between our house and the hospital, and I rummaged through my mother's dresser drawers until I found her swimming suit.

Dusk descended and the halls were eerily quiet as we rode the elevator up to my father's floor. Tyler stood nose to nose with the closed door, and Brennan punched the fourth floor button, smugly smiling.

"Grandpa's room is the first one on the right after we get off the elevator," I said. "This is a hospital. You need to be quiet. Other people are sick. And so is Grandpa. He will be in bed with an IV in his arm and an oxygen mask on his face. His tummy still hurts, so you need to be gentle."

They nodded solemnly. After all, they were both quite comfortable with hospitals and illness.

As soon as the elevator doors opened, they leaped out and sprinted down the hall, Brennan in front of Tyler, his long legs leading the way.

My parents told me later that as we approached the room, Dad said, "What is all that noise? It sounds like Brennan!" Seconds later, Brennan burst into their room, shouting, "Hi, Grandpa! Surprise!"

Grandpa let out a big belly laugh, throwing back his head and holding his pillow to his stomach to staunch the pain. My parents typically didn't like surprises, but this one they laughed about for months.

The next morning in the pool, Mom stood in the shallow end, throwing the boys the beach ball and laughing as they dove and splashed about. Mission accomplished. When we returned home that night, the boys hunted for Easter eggs. Brennan stayed well, and I was glad that we could provide my parents some respite and entertainment at such a stressful time.

*　*　*

Dad's second surgery, a lung resection for lung cancer, hit him hard. Once again, all four of us siblings arrived from four different states, carving out our roles. The pain management, uncertainty of the lymph node biopsies, and the incredibly long days waiting for the chest tubes to stop draining to seal off the air leak were my territory. But I too had to go home. It was Brennan's sixth birthday, he was still on treatment, and he had a nagging unwellness and elevated liver enzymes after a strep infection. I also had grant reviews due and my own research grant deadline. And Tyler needed dental surgery.

Brennan had finished his first year of kindergarten and was home when I arrived. He complained of stomach pains and body aches, he looked pale and lethargic, and he spent much of his day on the couch.

"Maybe if you go outside and get some sunshine you will feel better," I said.

"I can't, Mom. I don't feel good."

I felt guilty for leaving my parents, and I struggled with a lack of patience at home. Guilt was not a common feeling for me. Typically, if I wanted to be helpful I found a way to tend to everyone else's needs. But now guilt dripped like a leaky faucet, running a river beneath the surface of my life and draining away my precious reserves. I tried to balance the see-saw of needs, all with an expectation of positive goodwill. I hashed out my internal struggle in my journal, noting that Mom and Dad were immobilized by this second surgery, the painful and agonizingly slow recovery, and the cancer diagnosis. It was hard for me to be back home while they managed in the hospital without an advocate.

I had come to expect the unpredictability of Brennan's treatment. But the constancy of my son's and then my father's crises that winter, spring, and summer meant that I was always on call. The cumulative load of caregiving escalated my stress. And yet I don't know if, given the chance, I would have done anything differently.

* * *

Thankfully, my talk in San Francisco was sandwiched in between Dad's surgeries. We couldn't leave him alone, so my twin brother generously offered to fly home from California to be with Dad so Mom could fly out with Duane and the boys and Beth on the day of my talk. We were grateful to Jerry; it meant that we could relax and spend a few extra days enjoying San Francisco and Carmel after my talk.

I was already at the conference, waiting for everyone at the hotel. It was less than an hour before the talk, and they still hadn't arrived. Without cell phones, I had no idea what delayed them.

Suddenly they burst into my room, tumbling over each other to get through the door.

"We're here!" Brennan announced, followed by an exaggerated, eye-rolling, "Finally!"

"We sat on the tarmac for two hours," Duane said as he plopped the bags down in the corner.

"They wouldn't let you off?"

"No, we had already pulled away from the gate."

Brennan crawled into my bed and pulled the covers up to his neck. I sat down next to him, glancing at the red clock digits. They crisply clicked to 2:35.

"I know you are tired, but the talk starts in twenty-five minutes," I said. "Do you want to change before we go?"

"I don't want to go."

"But that's what you came out for," I said, suddenly aware that this had been my agenda, not his.

"I'm too tired."

"I know. It must have been an exhausting trip." I watched him finger the blanket edge. I toyed with the idea of letting him skip the talk. Two more minutes ticked by on the clock beside me. I heard the others shuffle around the room, the bathroom door snapping shut several times.

Suddenly, I blurted out, "How would you like to stand up on stage with me in front of 5,000 people?"

Brennan leaped out of bed and boldly announced, "Let's go!"

I glanced toward the suitcase still sitting in the corner and then turned to open the door, ignoring the dress shirt and pants tucked neatly inside. Everyone scurried out, following Brennan and me down the elevator and across the courtyards and streets. The two of us walked hand in hand into the convention hall to the front row of reserved seats.

"When do I get to come up on stage?" Brennan asked.

"When I tell you to or motion for you," I replied, having no idea how this was going to play out. He seemed content with the unplanned plan.

A friend did some quick energy therapy with me in a small room at the back of the convention center hall, her hands circling above and around my torso and head to clear blockages and channel positive energy from the universe. I took a deep breath and walked up on stage.

For fifty minutes I told the story of how the nurses caring for

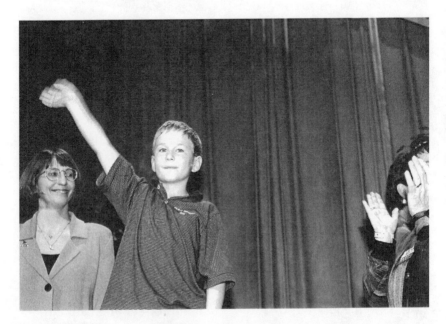

Author and Brennan, Oncology Nursing Society, San Francisco, 1998.

Brennan and our family empowered us to move forward on our journey, encouraging us through storms and rocky seas and celebrating with us as we charted our way through unfamiliar waters. "Sara is the gentle wind behind our sails," I said, "nurturing our confidence and our resilience." It felt so good to reconnect with a community of 5,000 mentors, colleagues, friends, and students.

As I ended the talk with slides of Brennan's artwork from that first year flashing onto the three huge screens, Brennan bounded up the steps to the stage. I had forgotten to signal him! The executive director, sitting next to me at the podium, promptly stood up and pulled out her chair for him to climb up on. Brennan beamed, standing as tall as me, waving his outstretched arm, high above his head, back and forth, back and forth.

He accepted all of the applause.

CHAPTER 18

Can't Escape Cancer

Caelhan died that September, eight months after her bone marrow transplant. Her parents, recently separated, stood together in a receiving line at the church, smiling and hugging those of us grieving her loss. I had come across her obituary in the newspaper the night before.

Duane and I sat in the church pew, surrounded by the same oncology nurses and physicians treating Brennan. We watched videos of Caelhan in her healthier days, smiling as she climbed out of the swimming pool, waving good-bye on her first overnighter. Normal kid stuff. Her mom and dad took turns telling stories at the front podium. They didn't cry; we did.

"Hi, Mom!" Caelhan would say cheerily every morning as she bounded down the stairs. Years later, I could still imagine her enthusiasm, her lightness, despite her weight gain, weakness, and advancing disease. I tried to forget the image of her on the day of the heme-onc picnic that July, when she had sat at the picnic table surrounded by the nurses who had cared for her before she went to the university for transplant. I regretted that I hadn't talked to her then. *She has people around her*, I had rationalized at the time. *She doesn't really know me. What would we talk about other than how she's feeling?*

In reality, it was too hard for me. I felt uncomfortable. I would eventually learn that when we don't know what to say, when we avoid others because of our own discomfort, it's because we fear getting too close to our own emotions.

I cried through the entire service, unable to stifle audible sobs. I cried for Caelhan, whose strength and beauty accompanied her through her last days. I cried for her parents, who lived with cancer or the fear of cancer for nine years and still lost their daughter. And I cried for Brennan, for what he had to endure, praying that he remained relapse-free and that his future promised joy. And I cried for us, his parents, who faced an uncertain future, never knowing but always hoping. A year and a half of tears spilled forth in that hour.

* * *

When I told Brennan that Caelhan had died, he nodded sadly. At six years old, he either didn't know what to say, didn't really remember her, or chose not to dwell on it. We never talked about her again.

He did talk about Max. Max was a new kid in first grade who had just moved back to Minnesota after living in Europe for several years.

"Max fell off the slide at school today," Brennan reported as I chopped vegetables for dinner. "Well, a bunch of kids did, but Max is the only one who got hurt."

"Max got hurt on the roller slide? What happened? How was he hurt?"

"I don't know," he said and then he moved on to talk about other events of his school day.

The following month, Brennan and I were at the hospital when he mentioned that Max was there for surgery.

"Really? Should we stop by to see him?" I don't know why I thought he might want visitors. I made a quick phone call to the room from a hospital phone to ask if it was okay if we stopped by.

The bright October sun shined through the picture window overlooking the city in Max's room. He was in bed, hooked up to several IVs and an infusion pump, looking at either a car or sports magazine. His dad stood when we walked in.

"Hi, Max!" Brennan announced.

"Hi."

Max looked up and made eye contact with Brennan and then turned back to his magazine.

"Hi, I'm Brennan's mom," I said as I held my hand out to Max's dad. "We just finished a talk and we're on our way back to school. We thought we would stop by and say hello." How trite that sounded;

my words echoed in the cavernous unease. I half-turned back to the door, and then looked at Brennan, who had just asked Max what he was reading.

"They just hung his IV," Max's dad said, seemingly uncertain of what or how much to say.

I had no idea what they knew about Brennan or his leukemia or my nursing background. I caught snippets of "surgery," "treatment," and "just diagnosed last Friday." Friday was six days ago, and it had been six weeks since the incident on the slide. What was he being treated for?

Max and Brennan started talking about what Max was missing at school.

"I have a tutor," Max said. "She comes here to the hospital."

"You have to do schoolwork in the hospital?" Brennan asked, his eyes wide. He had asked me a few times if we could go back to the hospital to stay "because it was so much fun." He was never there long enough to have to do schoolwork.

"Can you concentrate on homework?" I asked, turning my attention to the boys.

"Sort of." Max shrugged.

His mom later told me how hard it was to prod, push, and nag just to get Max to take a bath and his meds. Doing homework must have felt insurmountable when neither parent nor child had the energy for or saw the purpose in facing math, problem solving, or learning to read. I felt a sad camaraderie with them.

"How long are you going to be here?" I asked Max.

He looked up at his dad.

His dad said something that implied they weren't sure or that it depended on how quickly Max healed from the surgery.

I must have eventually asked, because by the time we left I knew that Max had a soft tissue sarcoma, a cancer that was discovered in his abdomen when he didn't heal properly or recover completely after his fall from the slide.

The IV they had just hung was his chemotherapy. But it was the urinary catheter that was the most troublesome for him, his dad said, and would be a continuing annoyance throughout his treatment. No wonder he seemed hesitant to see his new friend.

"Well, that was unexpected," I said to Brennan as we walked back to the car.

"So Max has cancer, too," he replied.

* * *

"What's the prognosis?" I asked Brennan's oncologist the following week after we told him about Max.

He listened to Brennan's lungs and then looked at me. "Not good."

I waited, watching him.

"Around 20, maybe 30 percent."

I didn't have the courage to ask how long Max might live.

* * *

It would be six more weeks before Max returned to class.

"Max's back!" Brennan said as he walked into the classroom that cold December day and saw a weak-looking but smiling Max seated at a table surrounded by seven or eight of his classmates, all of them excitedly chatting at once.

"How is it going?" I asked his mom, who was standing off to the side watching.

"Oh," she sighed, "better, I guess. There's so much to do. He's only off treatment for four days and I have to...."

I tuned out the details and focused on the wrenching feelings within my gut as I stood next to this mom who was so overwhelmed.

"Are you working?" I asked after a long pause.

"I was trying to keep up, but I can't, really. I have people to cover for me for a while."

The next month she told me that she and her husband were considering whose job took priority and how to trade off work roles and prioritize the bills.

"I didn't see you when you came into the hospital," she said. "My sister came to town, and I was so glad she did, because I could barely get out of bed. I slept for ten hours straight!"

"I did the same thing," I said, "a month after Brennan's diagnosis."

We nodded together as we watched the kids, not seeing anything beyond our grief.

* * *

The following day, the same child life specialist who had come to Brennan's kindergarten class a year before came again to explain to the kids what cancer was and wasn't. I had come to drop Brennan off at school but stayed to listen at the back of the room. Brennan sat in the front row on the floor next to Max.

"Now, we know that you can't catch cancer from each other. It's not like a cold or a flu virus," Vicki explained. "And we know that Max got hurt on the slide way back at the start of school, but that injury didn't cause the cancer, either."

A buzz went around the room. Many of the kids nodded their heads. The teachers had talked to them, intent on allaying misconceptions and fears.

Vicki went on to explain how Max was getting his treatment and what to expect. He already was bald and had missed two months of school, so that part didn't surprise them. When she showed them the port-a-cath site with an IV tube hanging out of the mannequin doll on her lap, Max and Brennan instantaneously sat up on their knees and turned around to face the class. They pulled up their white school shirts with both hands, puffed out their pale tummies, and showed off the bumps under the skin on their chests, smirking proudly.

Then Brennan leaned over to Max. "Hey, yours is on the left," Brennan said. "Mine is on the right."

* * *

Sometime during the next few days, Max's mom stood next to me before class and whispered, "The primary tumor is shrinking … and so are the metastases in his lungs. The chemotherapy is working."

"That's great news," I said, happy that she would share this with me and also aware that concrete, measurable results gave us all hope.

"After we told Max," she said quietly, "he asked what Heaven was like and what would have happened if the tumor hadn't responded."

I turned to her with a sad, sympathetic whimper. I could only hope that knowing I shared in her suffering and had compassion for her plight helped her feel a little less alone.

* * *

At a hospital-sponsored parent support group that fall, one of the child life specialists had told the group of twenty or so parents that "how well a child copes is not associated with the severity of the illness." This was very consistent across the research, she added. *But then*, I wondered, *what does determine how well a child copes with illness?* It seemed intuitive to me that children take their cues from their parents. And yet each family is different, and how families cope also depends on their past experience and their expectations.

According to theories on family resilience, families who have resources and support adapt better to illness. They get assistance with tasks, they feel less alone, and they find meaning in the illness. Children too tend to cope better when their family shows them love and security and when they talk about the illness and its effects, listen to and respect the child's feelings and concerns, focus on the positive, and address and solve problems when they arise. Children learn and grow from adversity, as adults do, and they need opportunities to show their strengths and independence, to become confident and competent, even when ill. But that's a long list to strive for! Especially when parents are just trying to get through each day.

After the visit from child life, Ella, another of Brennan's classmates, started asking her mom questions. That's when her mom told me that Ella had had retinoblastoma as a baby—though Ella didn't know it. She just knew that she had only one eye because of the surgery she'd had at birth. And it wasn't obvious to anyone in the class; her replacement eye looked very natural.

"We never told her she had cancer," Ella's mom explained to me one morning after we dropped the kids off for school. "We're from Spain. They don't talk about cancer there." And then she added, "We believed we were doing the right thing."

As Ella's mom struggled with how much and what to tell her six-year-old daughter, I contemplated the odds of there being three children with cancer in a classroom of twenty-one kids.

* * *

"There is something really unique about kids with cancer," my graduate student had said. "They are the future philosophers of the world, the deep thinkers."

Only later did I wonder if they were born with this unique insight or if they acquired it in response to the experience of having cancer. Caelhan's parents had talked of her uniqueness—her energy, insight, and maturity for her age. Ella's mom talked of her daughter's impatience with the mundane and frustration with a lack of stimulation. "She needs to be striving for something. She needs a purpose." Max questioned the value and purpose of everything he was expected to do. He just wanted to be outside with his friends.

Brennan had this "Zen being" that I labeled after we watched videos of him when he was three, before diagnosis. I wrote in my journal, "I need to pay attention and not brush off his concerns. He's usually right. He just knows."

The same week that Max returned to school, Brennan and I lay in his bed together after practice for the Christmas program at church.

"I wish I were Jesus," he said, out of the blue.

"Why?" I asked, turning back to him after reaching for a book from his book shelf.

"Because then I could rule the world."

"That's a lofty goal," I said as I smiled at his ability to think big and to have the energy and motivation to dream. After all, cancer wouldn't always rule our world.

I didn't think to ask him what he would change.

* * *

The following spring, Duane and I took our first trip without the boys. We ventured to Paris for six days, confident that Beth and Laurie could handle things while we were gone. Brennan was in his third and final year of treatment.

After visiting picturesque Sainte-Chapelle, with its dramatic vaulted ceilings encircled by intensely illuminated and gilded stained glass windows, we walked across the street into the vast, dark dampness of Notre Dame Cathedral. A priest dressed in white robes chanted in Latin at one of the altars while visitors shuffled quietly about observing the intricate stone architecture, engravings, and statues. Pillar candles sat on pedestals in alcoves, glowing like beacons direct to the heavens. Without hesitating, I fumbled in the semi-darkness in my purse and dropped a euro into the cup with a clink, then lit a candle in the middle of a dark grouping. I wanted it to outshine all of its neighbors.

"Let him live," I prayed. "Please get Brennan well." And we walked quickly out in silence.

CHAPTER 19

Decisions, Decisions

"How many more back medicines do I have to get?" Brennan asked as we drove home after his intrathecal treatment that spring.

I calculated the schedule through to the following March. "Four more."

He groaned as we pulled into the garage.

"How are you feeling?" I asked, thinking that it had gone better that day. He didn't have a headache, he hadn't thrown up, and we were home before noon. On bad days, he would vomit afterwards or get headaches so bad that he couldn't tolerate any light or stimulation for hours, and we would be in the darkened hospital room until mid-afternoon. We had switched anesthetics back to the Propofol and added an IV pain med.

"I just wanna go inside." He leaned his head back and sighed.

I wondered if the treatments were getting harder for him because he knew what to expect. He also knew the end was in sight, but he had to persist.

If he were a girl, he'd be done with treatment. Boys needed an additional year of systemic chemotherapy to prevent relapse in the testicles; the inclusion of an extra year of intrathecal chemotherapy, however, gnawed at my rational mind. Intrathecal chemotherapy specifically treated central nervous system (CNS) disease, and boys didn't have higher rates of CNS relapse that I knew of.

I might have been rationalizing or defending the scientific process, but I reassured myself that the oncologists and researchers had thought this decision through very carefully, over several years, before launching the clinical trial. In fact, several years after Brennan completed treatment, I would sit in on these committee meetings and complain along with my colleagues about the laborious and slow progress of moving clinical trials forward. Everyone meticulously belabored and debated every hypothesis, every patient characteristic, every outcome. I knew that only one or two conditions could be tested in each study, and it took years to accrue the several thousand children needed to get enough statistical power to determine the significance of the findings. Only recently have studies begun to address survivor quality of life and cognitive deficits in children receiving intrathecal chemotherapy without cranial radiation. Living well after cancer is a relatively new concern for researchers, now that more children are surviving.

While Brennan was on study, more than the expected number of children on triples developed seizures and cognitive problems with organization, concentration, attention, and academic ability, especially in abstract math. These effects on executive function had unexpectedly increased after treatment ended. Children under age five at diagnosis were at greatest risk because of their growing brain.

I mulled the options over and over. *Well, he was* almost *five*, I reflected, hoping for the best or trying to ignore the risk. Even though Brennan hadn't experienced seizures and wasn't exhibiting any obvious deficit, the risk was real. If boys didn't have any higher rates of CNS relapse than girls, would stopping intrathecals at two years reduce or prevent cognitive late effects, outcomes that might affect their self-esteem and quality of life? I contemplated dropping just the intrathecals from Brennan's last year of treatment. But that would require taking him off study. There was no safety, just best guesses.

While I was questioning Brennan's treatment, another clinic family we had become friends with was questioning whether to stop treatment early. Although Patrick had been eleven at diagnosis and was on a different treatment plan, we often were in clinic at the same time, and we shared the same nurse.

"Why would you stop Patrick's treatment early?" I asked his mom and dad, who always came to his treatments together.

"He starts high school in the fall, and we want him to have more energy," one parent said, and the other added, "We want him to enjoy his high school experience."

"Is he on a clinical trial?" I asked, thinking of what happens to the data analysis when a subject drops out of a trial.

"No, he didn't fit any of the criteria when he was diagnosed. They are treating him with the standard schedule from the previous trial."

I nodded, thinking of how this might influence their decision and if it would have changed mine. If Brennan wasn't on a clinical trial, would I be making different choices?

As a parent, I understood their motivation. My primary goal was my son's safety, survival, and future health. I wondered, though, if I could do it. Would I have the courage to take my son off of his life-saving treatment, even if he wasn't on a clinical trial? His treatment was our security blanket, tethering us to an imaginary lifeline. If we stopped just the intrathecals and he relapsed—at all, ever—could I live with my decision? On the other hand, if we continued on through three years and two months as scheduled, and he ended up with cognitive or neurologic deficits, would I feel responsible knowing there was a chance I could have reduced the severity of these effects? I dreaded any long-term cognitive effects, but, I rationalized, he would only know what he was capable of, not what he was missing. And because we hadn't done neuropsych testing at diagnosis, we would never really know for sure if any discrepancy was a direct result of treatment.

I thought about this decision for *months*. What were the chances of the leukemia relapsing in his central nervous system or of his experiencing lasting cognitive effects after two years of intrathecal chemotherapy? Would one more year really make a difference, either way? I went back and forth, questioning and answering myself. If Brennan was going to stay on the trial, he had to get the spinal chemotherapy. It was a package deal. I considered the greater good for all and what they would learn from this study.

In retrospect, I should have just asked his oncologist and shared my concerns. Instead, I struggled alone. I knew that I had to make the decision that felt right to me. I didn't want someone brushing off my concern, minimizing it, or blankly reassuring me. I didn't know who would take me as seriously as I did myself.

I tend not to look back once I make a decision, especially one I have thought through thoroughly or can't undo. I had to trust that keeping Brennan in the study was the best decision at the time.

I slid the idea into a conversation with Duane when we were talking about Patrick's decision. Duane's lack of challenge made me feel I was either on the right track, the track felt right to both of us, or that this was my decision, to be made alone. I didn't ask him whether or not he would support me in it. I expect that he never really knew the depth of my dilemma.

I kept Brennan on the trial. I couldn't convince myself to take him off. If he relapsed, most likely it would be in the central nervous system or testicles, and I would never forgive myself. His first chance for a cure was now. Survival was more important.

✳ ✳ ✳

Years later, the research would conclude that there were no benefits from either of the more aggressive treatments, the triples or the thioguanine. In fact, there was a higher rate of early bone marrow relapse in some children receiving triples. And the toxicities were significant enough to warrant new clinical trials without triples and with modified doses of thioguanine. Brennan still may be at higher risk for cognitive deficits from the intrathecal triples, or future liver problems as a result of the thioguanine and liver VOD, but no one knows what the long-term effects might actually be.

When he was fourteen, Brennan chose not to participate in follow-up studies that documented the cognitive and metabolic late effects of the children who had participated in his clinical trial. The studies required time and commitment and overnight hospital stays. By then, he just wanted to be a normal kid. As hard as it was to let the opportunity go, I let him choose. Knowledge was at stake then, not survival.

✳ ✳ ✳

It was sometime in early summer, when we were playing outdoor mini-golf together, that Patrick's parents told us they had decided to stop Patrick's treatment. He was feeling better, stronger, and they felt optimistic. I trusted that they, too, had made the right decision for them. We lost touch after both boys came off treatment.

CHAPTER 20

The Last Lap

Brennan's final year of treatment wasn't any less hectic, but we at least knew we were on the last lap. After a brief winter respite, Brennan developed six weeks of ear infections with recurring strep (necessitating another out-of-town emergency room visit), parvovirus/Fifth's disease (requiring another blood transfusion for anemia), a cracked clavicle from a bicycle fall (a major adaptation for an active seven-year-old), bronchitis—again—and exposure to chicken pox in our carpool (requiring a painful immunoglobulin shot and cautious wariness for twenty-one days over the holiday season). In between, Duane's father moved to a nursing home, and I somehow wedged in four speaking engagements, one of them to Japan. I was awarded tenure and entrance as a fellow into the Academy of Nursing that year. If I hadn't recorded it in my resume, I wouldn't have remembered.

It felt as if we had acclimated to a higher level of stress, as if climbing to a higher altitude. We had started out focused on our own self-preservation, on survival. As we learned the terrain and the road map, we learned to pace ourselves and to prepare for anything and everything.

I was a bit surprised that summer, though, when the pediatrician suggested a CT scan to evaluate Tyler's headaches. He had no nausea or vomiting or visual symptoms, but the headaches had persisted for three months.

"We should just be sure," the doctor said. "Given his brother's history."

The headaches had started in the spring, around Tyler's fourth birthday. Four. That was how old Brennan had been when the leg

158

pains started. I agreed to the CT scan, even though it meant radiation exposure to Tyler's growing brain.

Would I ever let go of the fear? I had spent three months analyzing Tyler's headaches, keeping notes on his diet, activity, sleep, and allergies. Had he gotten a concussion when he fell on the hill and scraped his cheek from his mouth to his eye? I had taken him to the pediatrician twice, risking the label of "overanxious" mother and losing another half-day of work. I tried to remain logical and composed. But in those wee morning hours, those very imaginative and creative hours when subconscious fears surface, I acknowledged that perhaps, just perhaps, because we were vulnerable, Tyler might have cancer, too. One family on the pediatric listserv I had joined had two boys with ALL, diagnosed two years apart. Another family had a daughter with neuroblastoma and a son with ALL.

A few days after we went in for the scan, I answered the phone on the first ring.

"I have the results from Tyler's CT scan," the voice said, absent of any reassurance. "The scan came back normal."

"Can you send me the report?" I wanted more data, more specifics. The voice was just telling me the conclusion without the supporting evidence.

"It just says 'normal.'"

"Oh, okay," I said quietly. I rallied a perky "Thanks!" before hanging up.

I was relieved—a little. Even conclusive evidence couldn't replace the feeling of vulnerability, the knowing that is forever etched in a parent's mind when one child has cancer.

I later deduced that Tyler's headaches were stress-related, with spring pollen and tree allergies frosting the tension at home. Our part-time sitter, who filled in when I taught in the evening and worked on Saturdays, was a good match for Brennan's intensity, but her energy overwhelmed sensitive Tyler. He was the single family member who could, refreshingly, put feelings before thinking. He would lightly touch my arm and ask, "How are you, Mom?" I would smile, reassure him, and hug him. Later that year, after the headaches resolved, he began to sometimes instruct me at bedtime, "Hold me like a baby," as he curled up alongside my beating heart.

Stress in two- to four-year-olds hasn't been studied. Only a handful of studies assess sibling responses to cancer, and they include only older children, those who can fill out forms, explain how they feel, or share their perceptions of how life has changed within their family. I fell into the same trap. Brennan was verbal. Tyler was quiet. And Tyler didn't draw.

Many years later, Tyler would search the literature for published papers on sibling responses to cancer for a college class on family communication. "There isn't much there," he said, shrugging. "I left you a copy of the paper I reviewed on your chair."

What he found in that thirty-page systematic review by Long and Marsland was that there is great variability in how families adjust to cancer and it depends on their "existing family functioning, marital quality, and parenting."

I hope he was reassured that most children with cancer, and their siblings, do not differ psychologically from their peers in the long run. They admit to feeling tension, loss, fear, confusion, powerlessness, and isolation shortly after diagnosis. Their world as they know it has changed dramatically overnight. But over time the kids adapt.

At twenty-one months old, all Tyler knew was that Brennan wasn't home and he had no one to ride scooters or eat lunch with. So he stopped playing and eating. He sat on the window seat, watching the traffic go by, shuffling his matchbox cars from one parking spot to another. I wrote in my journal that it took six weeks for Tyler to reestablish trust and to break out of the acute loss that he didn't know how to share with us.

Later I would read that most children overcome the initial anxiety and stress *if* their family learns to be flexible, adaptable, and supportive. But what does that really mean? And how did I know if our marriage and our family functioning were capable of getting us through without adverse outcomes in the end? I've tried to see it through Tyler's eyes, how we did as parents. Adapting didn't feel conscious to me. I was more like the Roadrunner continuously evading Wile E. Coyote, trying to outsmart and outpace the stressors. I just kept going and going. There was little time to pause, reflect, and reevaluate.

I've looked for clues in pictures and journal writings, sometimes surprising myself that, yes, I was there for them and I did, on occasion, talk to each of them about how they were feeling. Maybe not often enough and certainly not always when they needed me most and I was distracted. Accepting my limitations, past and present, is part of my letting go.

I have several friends and colleagues who study family coping and resiliency in the face of cancer, in both adult and childhood illness. I've advised on the conceptual models, pored over their research findings and publications, and even coauthored some. But living with cancer is a lot more complicated than studying it.

In theory, resilient families adapt and change. "Becoming a cancer family" means living as normally as possible, accepting that life will never again be the same, understanding what you have to do, and accepting what you cannot change. Each family finds their own way. Another parent described the experience years later as a "getting through" time of life. She and her husband had pushed forward, "like oxen leading the cart, each of us pulling our own load."

Our own rhythm felt more back and forth, a your turn/my turn approach to pulling the cart forward. I don't know that our roles ever quite felt balanced to me, but Duane was always there for back-up. Health was my territory; I took the lead. We didn't talk about the process or our responses; we fell into our independent and introverted ruts, doing what we felt we needed to at the time. Nonverbal communication had always ruled our interactions, and wishing it otherwise would have been unrealistic. So much history wrapped us in our cocoons.

There is strength in working side by side for a common goal and not getting wrapped up in each other's agendas. It worked for us. We survived because we focused on our strengths, on what was working, which was more productive than ruminating on deficiencies and shortcomings, which we all have.

Early on, I thought that families just moved on when treatment was over. I would later see that the patterns of communicating and interacting established during a long illness continue to weave their way into family dynamics. On one family trip, we let Brennan make many of the decisions about what to do, where to eat, and how to handle schedule changes. It bothered me afterwards that we didn't consult each other or take turns in making choices, but the vacation went smoother when Brennan was happy. He thrived on leading, and the rest of us didn't really want to do the legwork and planning that he expected. It was only later that I considered the idea that others in his life might not be so compromising.

* * *

Patrick's mom had encouraged me several times to join an e-mail listserv for parents of children with ALL. Once I did, I eagerly awaited posted updates. As I became more comfortable with the group, I reassured one concerned father, new to the vicissitudes of treatment, that his daughter's fluctuating counts were to be expected. "Don't read too much into the day-to-day changes," I advised. "Look for the bigger trends over time."

These were families, like ours, who one week navigated crises and in the next celebrated counts coming up, milestones passed in the road map, and time spent together outside of the hospital. These informed, compassionate, and caring parents generously shared their experiences and gave me support, encouragement, and reassurance, even when I didn't know I needed it. I gained perspective and gratitude through this new community. Some parents lingered after their child came off treatment, but most moved on to the survivor's listserv. I eventually lost touch with them over time, but I still think about those incredible kids and their awesome and resilient parents.

In October of that final year of treatment, as Brennan's broken clavicle healed in a sling, we flew to Phoenix to give the opening ceremony's keynote at the annual pediatric oncology nursing conference. I asked families on the listserv if they wanted to share some of their experiences with the nurses who cared for their families. They sent me pages and pages. Brennan stood up on stage next to me, voicing the children's contributions, while I spoke the wise words of their parents.

"I hate my pokeys!" said three-year-old Elsie.

"I feel so helpless when it comes to the procedures," said her mom. "The nurses treat her like the person she is…. They distract her from the negative things when I am at my wit's end."

"What bothers me most is the pain," said four-year-old Calli. "But the nurses help distract me."

"What bothers me the most is the fear of losing my daughter," said her mom.

"What bothers me most about having leukemia is that it is annoying to be treated differently by people," said fifteen-year-old John.

"And I'm bothered more by the long-term problems and the fear that the leukemia will not stay in remission," said his mom.

Other voices of the children, ages two to seventeen, resonated through the meeting hall.

"When I woke up, my mom was on the phone crying," said Alex. "Being five, I didn't quite understand, but I knew it was the worst thing that would ever happen to me."

Alex's mom acknowledged her own turmoil. "One part of me wanted to comfort and console my child, and another wanted to save his life."

"Will I ever play football again?" asked seventeen-year-old Daniel, who had just been awarded a college football scholarship.

"After leukemia, how can you be afraid of football?" replied his mom. She added, for the benefit of us less experienced parents, "When our kids have been sick, it's easier to hold them close than to let them go. But it is in letting them go, even just a little, that we let them convince themselves that they're going to be okay."

I added, "And that's how they convince their parents that we, too, will be okay."

I understood, although I was a long way from letting go.

* * *

My greatest effort during Brennan's final year of treatment was to let go of my expectations. I had come to accept the uncertainty of treatment and to trust my family's ability to adapt to whatever got tossed our way. And now I had to release my attachment to any particular outcome. Letting go, even a little, allowed me to reach out to others. We might have cancer in our family, but other families were living with it too.

Community became important to me. Sharing and being a part

of the bigger universe of families gave me perspective and healing. It was these moments of connection, and living with compassion, that made the aloneness and uncertainty of the "what next" bearable.

As we approached our final lap of treatment, reflecting on how far we had come and reaching out to others helped me to accept where we were and nudged me forward. I turned the calendar on a new year and a new millennium. March 2000, end of treatment, was just the flip of a few pages, the final jaunt through the long, twisted tunnel to get to the finish line.

Chapter 21

Celebrate!

March 2, 2000, was damp, chilly, and dreary, but we didn't care. It was Brennan's last intrathecal medicine, his last triples. And his final, end-of-treatment bone marrow aspirate, which left his hip hurting and his head aching with the familiar dizziness. It was a tough climax, but we were at the top of the mountain. I struggled a bit with the ambivalence of it all. I wanted to be elated, to shout for joy, and yet I knew I needed to hang in there with him, subdued, as he endured. We had four more days of oral meds. *Then* he would be off treatment.

He politely posed for a picture from his recovery bed with his oncologist and nurse. It was a forced smile. He didn't want any cupcakes.

Four days later, nine friends came to his "off chemo" party. I savored their energy, enthusiasm, and joy as they burst into our house and plopped on top of each other in chairs in the family room, giggling, shouting, laughing joyously, and high-fiving Brennan, who wore a white polo shirt stamped with "3–6-00" and "end of chemo!" Even almost-five-year-old Tyler smiled as they shoved him over to make room for at least three others in his chair.

One friend made Brennan a heart-shaped ceramic plate painted with "Thank Heavens You're Well."

Yes, Charlotte, I thought, *exactly*.

Afterwards, Brennan asked me, "Can we celebrate every year?"

* * *

Finishing chemo wasn't exactly the end of the road for us, although it was the end of the road maps. Brennan wouldn't get his port-a-cath out until August, just in case he needed antibiotics or a blood transfusion, which meant regular clinic visits and blood tests, as well as trips to the ER or clinic for any fevers. Other parents on the ALL listserv had warned me that many kids get sick after treatment ends, which seemed to take parents by surprise. True to prediction, Brennan caught strep and a virus just as we ended our celebratory spring break trip in Phoenix.

The boys still chatted all the way home.

"I liked inner tubing on the river the best!" Brennan said.

"Me too!" Tyler echoed.

"And Camp Coyote!" Brennan went on, almost breathless. "And the two-story casita where we stayed. I liked sleeping on the first floor with Mom and Dad upstairs."

At the time, their level of excitement surprised me, but then I realized that most of our vacations had been with extended family since Brennan had gotten sick. It wasn't so much the warm and sunny location, or even being together alone as a family, but their newfound independence. How long had it been since we had loosened the reins? And how long had it been since Duane and I went golfing alone, without the boys? The other couple we were paired with on the golf course were so excited for us that they took pictures and later mailed them to us at our home.

A few weeks later, I typed in my journal:

> **Off treatment is fabulous!!!** *I still can't believe how quickly we put the whole experience behind us. Of course, it is integrated into our every cell and soul, but it's not on our conscious minds at all! I sincerely can't wait for every parent to experience the freedom and joy we have so graciously and appreciatively accepted this past month.*

I set aside any worries, at least for the moment. I even sent Brennan on a plane to New York City with a friend, where they met Duane and my friend's husband, who were working there that week.

Duane called one night after they had been to the Statue of Liberty, Times Square, and the Empire State Building. "He's so tired every night! All he wants for dinner is mac and cheese or room service. I can't get him to go back out."

Brennan got on the phone and added, in an exasperated tone,

"We had to walk everywhere, like eight miles! Dad wouldn't even take a taxi!"

I sympathized and smiled on the other end of the line. I didn't worry. It helped that his counts were great the day before he left, with an absolute neutrophil count over a record three thousand.

He had his first-ever sleepover the following weekend. He was tired, exhausted, even, but he wasn't the cranky and irritable kid on chemo. In fact, he seemed a different kid already. He was more affectionate, open with his emotions, and happier, with a more positive nature. He even spontaneously said, "I love you, Mom," something I hadn't heard without lots of coaching and cajoling those past few years (if ever). It wasn't just the physical benefit of coming off the chemo and prednisone; the change was immediate. I knew then that the weight of the world had been on his shoulders as he bravely, though not always willingly, did what he had to do to get through. It was like the little yellow bird had flapped his wings and flown off, because he could.

The next week was Tyler's fifth birthday and every cell in my body exhaled in relief.

* * *

By the end of treatment, Brennan had missed seven and a half weeks of chemotherapy because of illness and low counts and had an additional twelve weeks of reduced ("half-dose") chemotherapy. I calculated that over three years he'd missed 5 percent of his scheduled chemotherapy and received 8 percent at reduced doses. I never compared this to other children on the clinical trial. I really didn't want to know where he fit into the curve or how it might affect his survival statistically. Some things just couldn't be reduced to numbers.

"He's going to be fine," one of our oncologists said to me, intently but quietly enough so that I had to lean in to hear, as the end of treatment approached. I must have mentioned something about my fear of coming off treatment.

He's going to be fine. I repeated the words to myself over and over, implanting the prediction into my psyche. These five words carried me through the next five years, as long as I needed to keep reminding myself. The syllables cemented a bridge to our future, one I could walk across with anticipation and hope.

Coming off treatment is scary. Parents refer to treatment as the "chemo blankie." It's our security that the cancer is under control. Once the blanket is stripped off, our child's body is naked, vulnerable to the potential ravages of the one single cancer cell that might escape immune surveillance. Could we be sure they were all gone, completely eradicated in that three-year siege? Or were there some alive but hiding? Testing for minimal residual disease was just emerging as we came off treatment. It would eventually become routine, and although not conclusive for predicting relapse, it would be capable of detecting subclinical presence of leukemia cells.

Brennan wasn't tested, and I felt vulnerable to uncertainty. I had to trust.

"Is he in remission?" some people asked innocently.

I always hesitated. His liver enzymes were still higher than they should be, but the blasts in his bone marrow confirmed remission at 0.4 percent. "Yes, he's in remission, but he has been since day twenty-eight," I often replied—but then I had to explain, since he had had 1,200 days of treatment after going into remission. When I didn't have the energy, I simply said, "Yes." When silence followed, I felt inadequate, like I hadn't done my job.

"Is he cured?" others asked.

Cured? I wasn't sure when I would consider my son free of potential relapse. I expect I was supposed to feel reassured when some magic amount of time since diagnosis or time since the end of treatment clicked by, like the grandfather clock striking twelve—but the inconsistency and lack of clarity regarding when that should be annoyed me. Was the five-year mark people talked about calculated after treatment ended or after diagnosis?

Some experts considered children cured if they survived without any evidence of disease five years after diagnosis. That sounded like a long time, but it was less than two years away. Would I feel secure that soon? Others pointed to the five-year mark after treatment ended, which made more sense to my conservative, logical mind, especially since Caelhan had relapsed after four and a half years. Would I ever completely breathe a sigh of relief that my son was not at risk of relapse? To a researcher, 100 percent certainty isn't a real statistic. Some probability always exists.

At first, I was so elated to be off treatment I reassured everyone, including myself. Eventually, I found myself saying, "Yes, but," teaching others that although 80 percent of our children survive, the cost of treatment comes with consequences, the "late effects" that compromise their health and keep their parents vigilant. Yes, he was safe. For now.

* * *

Three months off treatment, Brennan stood on stage in front of almost 2,000 cancer caregivers in Washington, D.C., and said, "When I was four and a half I found out I had leukemia. Today is my birthday and I'm eight years old." The entire audience clapped, and then, as we watched from the stage, they stood as one, fanned out in front of us, and spontaneously sang "Happy Birthday." Brennan stood straight and tall, like a lightning rod grounded in his experience. I beamed up at him from my chair, alongside four other speakers. I knew that if I looked across that auditorium, filled with friends, colleagues, my family, and one of our oncologists, I would very unprofessionally lose it.

When they finished singing, Brennan smiled, thanked them, and went on with his talk. At the end he said, "What really helped me the most was having my family with me and believing in myself, knowing that I could get through it. Oh, and having basketball at the clinic was really great too. But most of all, I knew I could do it."

Brennan's eighth birthday symbolized a new birth, a new beginning. We could accept and honor the past; it had gotten us to where we were that day. We felt profound support in a world bigger than our own. We stood steady in time, trusting in the future, but planted firmly in the present, celebrating with joy.

Two weeks later Brennan and I drove two hours to Olivia, a small town in western Minnesota, to speak at an American Cancer Society Relay for Life event. When he found out that competitive events were planned and participants were camping overnight, he wanted to stay. We made it to midnight.

As dusk creeped in, Brennan leaned forward, seated

cross-legged on the black-topped high school track, listening intently to other stories of survival. Two of the other speakers, young adults, were sharing how cancer had interrupted their dreams and their plans and how they had leaned on family and friends to get through treatment and rely on their strengths. When it was time for the survivors' victory lap, Brennan glanced back at me, sitting behind him, and without a word, he jumped first in line

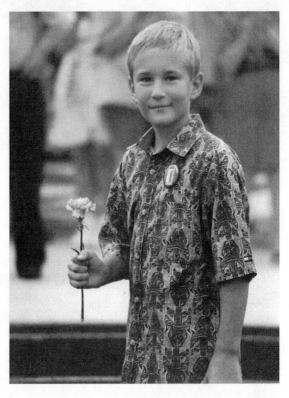

Brennan at the American Cancer Society Relay for Life, survivor's walk, Olivia, Minnesota, 2000.

and took the lead. He walked ahead of everyone else by half the length of the track. Halfway around, he turned and faced the camera, and me, confident in his victory.

PART III

The Decade After
Moving On

It's only when we can dwell in the places that
scare us that equanimity becomes unshakable
and we stop struggling with ourselves.
—Pema Chodron, *The Places That Scare You*

CHAPTER 22

Facing Fears

"Mom, could I have died?" Brennan asked me as I walked into his bedroom after just getting home from work. I was surprised to find him in bed. I quickly scanned him from head to toe, assessing for any illness. He was lying in bed reading *When Mom Has Cancer,* a book I was using for a research study. I had left it on the kitchen counter that morning.

I lay down next to him, our bodies seeping up the late-afternoon summer sun as we stretched ourselves out like the legs of a clothespin. I watched as his slim, eight-year-old fingers skillfully turned to the sixth chapter. I let my silence usher him on.

"It says here that the mom has breast cancer and that 10 to 20 percent of women die from it." He pointed to the paragraph as proof. "I had cancer, too. Could I have died?"

"Yes," I admitted quietly, with a hint of relief that we were finally talking about this reality. I looked up; his eyes stayed focused on the book. "Some children who get leukemia do die," I said. "That's why it's so important to start treatment as quickly as possible." I avoided pointing out that he was only a few months off treatment and relapse remained a real danger.

"She has a port-a-cath, too, but she only has to go in once a week for treatment. I had to go in every day some weeks!"

I couldn't tell if he was feeling pompous or envious. I hesitated. "Yes. That was a lot, wasn't it? Different cancers are treated with different medicines and schedules, but most people with cancer are treated with some type of chemotherapy because it kills the cancer cells. It also kills some healthy cells, which is why you—and this mom—lost your hair and had mouth sores and nausea. You need some time off in between treatments."

The teacher in me monopolized my intention. I struggled to put myself back into his world, to think about why he was asking these questions. Why was this so hard for me? Was I afraid he would shut down? I thought about the mothers with breast cancer and their children, the eight- to twelve-year-olds in the study. "She has children your age; I wonder what they are thinking."

"When she is done with treatment, will she live?" he said, more wondering than asking.

I didn't know if he was responding on behalf of the children in the study, asking if their mother would survive breast cancer or if he was identifying with the mother as a fellow cancer survivor and asking if he himself would live. I wish that I would have probed further, but he had just come off treatment. After three and a half years, I was so relieved to be thinking about living each day, reclaiming the childhood we had missed out on. It wasn't *his* reticence to face death, it was mine.

* * *

Brennan had surgery in mid–August to remove his port-a-cath. Sara handed it to us in a clear Ziploc bag. I tucked it away in a box, alongside his curly blond hair from his first haircut, his first baby tooth, and his childhood cancer survivor gold ribbon from the 1998 White House Christmas tree. I tossed the medication bin that had sat on top of the fridge for three years and eight months. We were free! Third grade here we come!

Before we knew it, Tyler had started kindergarten, our nanny Beth had left for medical school, and super-energetic Christopher had joined our family team, engaging the boys in after-school activities—football, baseball, basketball, tennis, and homework. We were six months off treatment, and we were moving on.

Third grade also brought crises for our small, close school community. In the midst of our celebrating and moving on, Max died.

Just five months earlier, at Brennan's first off-treatment oncology appointment, we had stopped by Max's hospital room. "Final Four is on. Want to watch?" Max motioned for Brennan to join him on the bed. Two sets of pale, skinny legs scissor-kicked the air as they lay on their stomachs, arms thrusting out to announce slick lay-ups and three-point swishes. Max's mother and I sat in chairs on the other side of the bed and solemnly talked of Max's recurring cancer. There wasn't much to say. The Midwest March day was gray and wet outside, and inside the air felt heavy with a resigned hopefulness, the clear liquid chemotherapy running on a timer into Max's bloodstream.

At Max's funeral service, the first week of school, Ella's mother told me that Ella, the other third-grade cancer survivor, had transferred to another school. She seemed relieved to have her daughter distanced from her unspoken history. I was glad to see her there, supporting Max's family and feeling as if she was still a part of our community. I felt a sense of closure. We could leave cancer behind now.

And then, that same year, tragedy struck two other school families. Brennan's friend's sister, a ninth grader, died suddenly after a brief respiratory illness during the holiday season. Surprised to see her name in the obituaries, I ran into the family room with the newspaper, where Brennan and a friend were playing a game on the floor.

"No, I didn't know his sister was sick," Brennan said. "That's too bad." He went back to playing Risk.

I carefully cut out Emily's picture from the *Star Tribune* and smiled back at her carefree grace, then tucked her obituary in a plastic sleeve in Brennan's school portfolio. To others this might seem inconsequential, as if her death were just another milestone event in elementary school—but it wasn't to me. For weeks I imagined her family and the healthcare team struggling to sort out the symptoms, to find a cause, and to treat it. Acutely labored breathing is frightening to experience and to watch. And to lose a child, suddenly, under any condition, was inconceivable. Or perhaps it was because I could imagine it that I felt it so profoundly.

And then Tyler's classmate's four-year-old sister was diagnosed with astrocytoma, a brain cancer originating in her spinal cord. Despite surgery, chemotherapy, and radiation therapy, Kami couldn't walk, and yet she still delighted in attending the same kindergarten classroom Brennan and Tyler had. The teacher, Molly, commented to me in the hall one day as she wheeled Kami back from assembly, "She has such a beautiful spirit. It's a joy to have her in class." Molly was the same teacher who had been able see Brennan's optimism through his prednisone outbursts.

We had Kami and her family over for dinner early on in her treatment. At one point, Kami, trying so hard to be like the other kids, lost her balance and tipped to the floor. Frustrated and crying, she curled up in a ball. Her mom stalwartly picked her up and gently wrapped her arms around her, whispering soothing reassurance as she caressed her daughter's shiny black hair. I paused in my cooking, watching this mom's strength and confidence—and her gentleness. After dinner, I cheered as Kami's two siblings chased our boys around the house, shouting orders and laughing out loud. *Just let them be kids*, my heart pleaded.

Kami lived for two years with progressive deterioration and intense family sacrifice and loving care.

There was so much cancer and so much death in one little school.

I vacillated between being supportive and caring and distancing myself as a form of self-protection. Brennan was off treatment, but he was still at risk for relapse. I still felt vulnerable. I was incredibly grateful for my son's life and yet despairing that these other children didn't live. These early lessons in death and grief and disability and loss had to have slithered into Brennan's psyche, too. How can you ignore your fears when they are mirrored back to you, over and over again?

* * *

Starting sometime after he came off treatment, and for years afterward, Brennan dreamt of death. His death. When I asked him to tell me more, he usually said, "I don't remember much, other than I died," or "I died falling off a cliff," or "I fell into a deep, dark hole." The dreams didn't seem unusual, except that his dying was consistent and persistent. Over the next ten years his dreams, or his memory of the dreams upon awakening, became more explicit. I never knew what to do with the information. I kept hoping that if he talked through them, they would eventually stop.

After one night of restless sleep, when he was around twelve, Brennan said, "It isn't like I wake up knowing I'm going to die. I see myself dead and then I wake up." He looked directly into my eyes, making sure I understood.

"That's unnerving," I said, sitting on the edge of his bed, trying to imagine what it would be like seeing your own body lying lifeless on the ground. I had always thought people woke up from dreams when they were in danger, before they actually died. I waited for more.

Silence followed.

"Tell me again how you died?" It felt better to have something specific to ask. But why couldn't I just ask him how the dream made him *feel*?

"Most of the time I get shot or attacked. Sometimes I'm in an alley and I get shot in the back or get caught in crossfire. Other times I face the perpetrator." He hesitated; I was looking at him quizzically, intrigued by his word choice. He was dissociated from any feeling, like an observer watching a movie. "But I always die. I see myself lying on the ground, not breathing, blood everywhere."

I wasn't sure what to make of the graphic finality. I had asked for specifics and he had circled back to the important message, seeing himself dead. I had left that fear dangling.

He would sometimes ask me to analyze his dreams. On four sequential nights one summer, he dreamed that he died in Boston. "What does that mean?" he asked the next morning at breakfast.

"I don't know," I said. "I don't know that the place is so important." I was more concerned by the pattern of his being a victim.

The dreams continued for years, although I was never quite certain of their frequency since he only talked about them occasionally, every few months.

When he was in his late teens, Brennan asked me about the detail in his dreams. "I notice everything, even the wrinkles on a person's face, the color of their eyes, and the make and model of the cars driving by."

"You're a detail guy," I said. "You notice these things in real life, so your subconscious processes them, too. I'm not a dream expert."

But I was intrigued. I later consulted a dream analysis, which said that dreaming of death meant change, new beginnings, and leaving the past behind. Of course, I paid attention to what I most wanted to hear—that the dreams meant a positive direction, a "moving on" kind of future. I needed time and distance to allay my concerns and to calm my son's fears.

"I'm not afraid of dying," he insisted over the phone while at college. "I think that's why I dream about death so much."

"It's a game," I suggested, relieved to know that he had at least considered his fears, even if he ruled them out. He was always so logical and analytical. "You play a game with life and a game with death. Strategy is your forte."

And then he told me about a dream in which he had flown to Paris to meet a publisher. They were having lunch in a café on Rue St. Honoré, and someone drove a car through the window. "I'm sitting with my back to them, but I know from past dreams that the car crashes into the restaurant and hits me, so I dive to the floor, as far from the impact as I can. It's totally a reaction. I don't have time to process things, which is why working it out in a previous dream helped me respond. I'm conditioned to think about self-preservation. I just act."

I thought back to those three years of my being in survival mode. Of course he had felt it, too.

He went on to tell me that in the dream he left the restaurant scene, unscathed this time, and walked into a local market on his way back to his hotel, only to be caught in an armed robbery. This time he was prepared, and he safely interrupted the hold-up. It wasn't until he was flying home and the plane depressurized and the oxygen masks didn't descend that he panicked. He had never confronted this problem and had no idea how to mechanically pry open the oxygen compartments. He died in his dream, along with everyone else on the plane.

He told me about the dream the next day. By then he had searched online and investigated how to get the oxygen compartments open, just in case he dreamt it again. "Maybe I am setting myself up for my next dream."

"Maybe you're setting the stage for your first novel."

He laughed lightly, not yet ready to move on.

"It takes a lot of time and energy to be prepared for everything that could possibly happen in life," I said. I couldn't tell if the game of outrunning death kept him engaged or if the dreams haunted him until he figured out a solution. This was the first time I'd seen his direct determination to conquer death in his dreams. What was his motivation? If he could figure out how to circumvent death through strategy, why couldn't he program his mind not to dream of death at all? If the dreams reflected subconscious fears, perhaps talking about them would bring them into awareness so that he could consciously let them go. But it had been thirteen years and he still dreamed.

He was like a samurai warrior, preparing for all the things that might go wrong, imagining and practicing his way out of any situation. Samurai use this strategy to stay cool and calculating in battle. Nothing surprises them because they have prepared themselves for everything.

But can we ever be prepared for death? Or cancer?

"It is a game," he eventually agreed. "I work out in my dreams how to stay alive and how to die."

"How is it that you always lose?" I asked.

"I don't lose. I win."

As I pondered his perspective on winning, I was reminded of a conversation we had late at night when he was sixteen and in high school. I had walked into the shadowy family room, lit only by the computer screen on his lap and the television across the room. I leaned over the back of the stuffed leather chair that he sat in sideways, his size fifteen feet clad in threadbare athletic socks, dangling in midair over the arm. He glanced up at me and then quickly flicked back to the screen on his lap. I watched him play his game in the dark—football, soccer, basketball, tennis, golf, one of those—it was always a sports game. The late-night show echoed from the television in the background. This twilight zone was our time, when his dad and brother slept.

"Hey, how's it going? What are you playing?"

He answered, and then suddenly, as if in defense of his passion for sports games, he blurted out, "I just can't get myself to play war games or violent video games where I know I'm going to die."

I nodded. He knew I detested guns. When he was six years old, he had come home from a comedy movie with a friend and said, "You wouldn't like it, Mom. The guy carried a 'you know what.'"

After a pause and the click of a few more plays with the computer arrow keys, he added, "If I do play, I hide to protect myself. Like behind a barrel or a wall. I just can't set myself up to be killed."

"Unlike Tyler," I said, and we both nodded, thinking of how his brother spent hours every day playing war games, dying and clicking himself back to life as he built his dynasties.

"You sometimes play *The Godfather* with Tyler," I reminded him, cringing at the images of shooting human beings in their homes and cars.

"Oh, that's easy to beat," he said, clicking another play on his computer.

"So winning is important."

He agreed.

The violence seemed less distressing to him than the vulnerability involved in putting himself at risk. He was happier playing sports, where losing didn't cost him his life.

I still don't understand, though, how he wins when he dies in his dreams. Perhaps it's because he allows himself another chance, a replay in his next dream. The will to survive motivates him to explore a solution. He's still in the game. He's got another chance.

* * *

Brennan's dreams of death were never about leukemia or illness, but they always involved something external—and random—happening to him. I could see how thwarting death in his dreams and video games was another way to prevail over vulnerability.

Figuring things out fosters a feeling of control. And feeling in control can be empowering, as long as it isn't an escape or defense. The Rev. Alla Renée Bozarth cautions in *Life Is Goodbye Life Is Hello* that holding on tightly to control can be a way to avoid feeling fear or any uncomfortable emotion, allowing feelings to simmer unannounced. "You need to feel the fear before you can release it," Bozarth advises. And since our natural tendency is to avoid our fears, we resort to control.

When Brennan came off treatment, he wrote for a class

assignment, "This event taught me how capable I was of doing things I didn't think I could do. It gave me confidence in myself because I had gotten through this whole thing … [it] taught me to believe in myself and to believe in my abilities to do things."

His mastery and confidence had come with practice, experience, time, support, and a positive outcome, a result he had little control over. He had learned resiliency while facing cancer, but did he know what he feared?

I thought it was death that Brennan feared. So I was surprised when I came across a paper he had written for his English class titled "My Greatest Fear: Europe on My Sixteenth Birthday."

I sat down, paper in hand. *This* was his greatest fear? His first trip to Europe? A fifteen-day family vacation in three countries? I leaned back on a stack of pillows on the window seat. He hadn't shared this paper or these feelings with me.

It wasn't the smoothest trip, I admit. Our connecting flight was canceled, Brennan fell asleep and forgot his birthday *Mad Men* DVDs under the seat in the airport, it took two hours to get the rental car in Geneva, and the roads to our hotel in Bern, Switzerland, were closed for the Euro Cup Fan Zone. But Brennan didn't mention these hassles in his paper. And he didn't say anything about being designated the chief navigator and German translator.

Duane and I had purposely paced activities on the trip, allowing time for hanging out as a family. We followed Brennan through the crowded Fan Zone, snapped pictures of him in front of the statue of Freddie Mercury (of Queen), played life-size chess and mini-golf in the park, and spent hours at the Duomo, checking out every dark corner inside and each spire and gargoyle outside in the summer mist. We jaunted through the Louvre during the day and raced down the Eiffel Tower stairs at night, trailing Brennan all the way. I wanted to take the boys into Notre Dame to light a candle and offer a decade-later blessing and thank you, but they didn't want to go inside, so we didn't.

As the trip progressed, Brennan became increasingly sullen and resistant. I attributed his frowns in pictures and his abject apathy during long walks as a response to itineraries that weren't his, being tired, and being sixteen. He was out of his comfort zone, in unfamiliar countries, facing new and novel experiences. Three months later, however, when he processed his feelings on paper, this is what emerged:

> *One of my least favorite things is change, or when I don't know where I am, where I'm going, or what I will be doing.... I wanted to have a fun, planned out trip, where all of our activities were laid out ahead of time. I always liked to know what would happen next, but in this new environment I was being forced to face my fear of lack of order, of uncertainty. I had no control anymore.... I was forced to follow my parents' every move, beat into submission by uncertainty.*

I set Brennan's paper in my lap and stared out the family room window, visualizing the streets of Bern, Menaggio, Milan, Venice, and Paris, and I sighed. The lack of structure had tripped him up. We had changed his environment, his routine, and his role, sweeping away order and stability. He could speak German but he couldn't grasp flexibility.

If uncertain vacation itineraries were so stressful to someone who thrived on order and predictability, what must it have been like to have cancer? Or was this defense a consequence to that experience, an ongoing attempt at control?

And that's when it struck me: Brennan wasn't afraid of death in his dreams, he was afraid of losing control.

CHAPTER 23

Wake-Up Call

Work ramped up the year Brennan finished treatment. I had five research studies underway, two of them testing aromatherapy and massage therapy in pediatric oncology and three testing massage/healing touch, acupuncture, and a cognitive behavioral therapy in adult oncology. I had competent and collaborative team members to manage day-to-day operations, recruit patients, run laboratory assays, and conduct interventions. I also had a dozen students working with me to complete their projects and theses using the data we were collecting.

It had been a decade since I had completed my doctoral degree, and integrative medicine was finally becoming accepted—and funded. In 1998, just two years earlier, the National Institutes of Health had established what would eventually become the National Center for Complementary and Integrative Health. This official designation as a center meant available funding for rigorous scientific research on the usefulness and safety of complementary and integrative health interventions. About the same time, new medical journals specific to complementary medicine and psychoneuroimmunology were being founded—perfect places in which to publish our findings and clinical advances. Integrative health had finally arrived.

The first spring after treatment ended, I participated in a research workshop for doctoral and post-doctoral nursing students in California. At the welcoming reception, a faculty colleague who held esteemed leadership positions at a major university and the National Institutes of Health walked directly up to me, stood inches from my face in her East Coast style, and announced, "Janice, I only have one regret—that I didn't spend more time with my boys. They are now seventeen and twenty." I was speechless. I had no idea why she was telling me this, at this time and in this setting. My boys were five and eight, and I couldn't really relate; all of my extra time seemed to be consumed with caring for them. I relished the thought of having free time! But the intensity of Ruth's message wormed its way into my psyche.

The next day at lunch I sat next to Mark, another faculty colleague, who shared captivating stories of spirit and transcendence in patients with cancer living in the Appalachian Mountains. What most struck me, however, was an acknowledgment unrelated to his work: "My youngest boy is now fourteen, and he doesn't want to spend time with me," Mark said.

I asked him what his son liked to do and whom he spent time with. Maybe this was normal! But the accompanying revelation startled me. Six years from now, when Brennan was fourteen, would he cringe at the thought of spending time with his mom? Just as I was trying to catch up on childhood, I was propelled into imagining him growing up and moving on.

I tucked away the milestone year and reflected, almost daily, about my role in my sons' lives. How old would Brennan be when he tired of chatting with me about school or when he stopped imploring me to "please do something with me"? I could never keep up with him, it seemed; he was an extrovert who craved entertainment and intellectual stimulation and who lived with three introverts.

Suddenly, time felt short. We were finally moving on with our life, rebuilding some sense of normalcy. To have Brennan slip away from me emotionally at age fourteen seemed so unfair.

I had a nagging feeling that if I wasn't careful, I could miss out on an important time as a family. And I started to recognize the difference between caring for my boys and connecting with them—right around the time I was struggling to keep up because of my health.

One particular day after school I could barely keep my head up without holding it in my hands. I was sitting with Brennan and Tyler at the kitchen table negotiating after-school activities.

"Let's play football or basketball," said Brennan. "You pick, Tyler."

"Either one," said Tyler, characteristically quiet and agreeable.

The weather was temperate and sunny, which would normally

draw me outside. "Can't we just play a game at the table?" I pleaded, feeling guilty that I couldn't provide the physical outlet Brennan needed. I wouldn't get Tyler to play without me. We compromised on an hour of Frisbee golf in the neighborhood, with trees and light-poles designating the holes. It took all of my energy to stay upright.

My immune deficiency and autoimmune conditions began a downward spiral. I frequently admonished myself to get my priorities straight, to find a better balance, and to realistically evaluate my own health limitations. Instead, I just kept putting one foot in front of the other. Then, one day, I realized I wasn't doing any one thing really well.

This was when my colleagues at the workshop reminded me that I also had limited time. My boys' childhood had been cut short, according to my expectations, and we were running to catch up to what we had missed. But I couldn't run anymore.

I again called my brother, Jerry.

"It's so hard to balance all the teaching, research, writing, and meetings," I told him. "And yet I don't know if I can let all my hard work go."

"Can you cut out the meetings?" he asked.

I smiled; he had suggested the same thing when I was debating whether to go back to work after Brennan first started treatment. "I don't think that's enough now."

"Can you get out of any classes?"

"I'm thinking of taking a semester off without pay," I said.

We talked about the logistics and consequences. Being an academic professor, he understood.

"But I'm also thinking long term," I said. "Can I keep doing this?"

And then I reminded him that my work was his investment too. Jerry had sacrificed his entire spring break to help me enter my research data and set up the analysis plan. I had flown out to his house in Tennessee, and we'd sequestered ourselves in his home office from morning to night for six days. He'd even forfeited half of his afternoon bike rides during that time to ensure we got everything done. And then he'd spent months afterwards writing the statistical software for the structural equation program he knew would work best for my data but wasn't yet developed for sale. I was incredibly thankful.

"Jerry, you should market this program!" I told him.

"Nah, I did it for you."

He even flew to Minnesota for my after-defense party. He showed up at the outdoor plaza an hour into the party, walked quickly through the door, caught my eye, and ran over, sweeping me off my feet and twirling me around, my skirt flying and his arms holding me secure. I was euphoric.

Jerry waved away my concerns about the sacrifices he'd made to help me. "Do what you need to do for yourself," he said after hearing me talk again about my lack of energy, my need to establish priorities, and my realization that the boys wouldn't be home forever. He didn't have children, but he took the time to understand how I felt.

I had choices. Not everyone does. I had continued to work during Brennan's treatment, mostly because I couldn't make decisions while in survival mode. Just as I emerged from that long, dark tunnel, Ruth and Mark shined a light. They showed me the way, and I am grateful.

* * *

I didn't rush change. It had to feel right, and I wasn't comfortable leaving work in the middle of projects. I devised a long-term plan to phase out my research and set up a consulting role that would allow me to work at home. I tossed the idea out to a few of my closest colleagues at meetings, who wholeheartedly supported me. It was like trying on a cloak and checking myself in the mirror. But I wasn't sure. How could I give up everything I'd worked so hard for, and for more than fifteen years?

I gave the decision time to percolate. Meanwhile, I was recruited for and offered an endowed professorship at another university in another state. I was honored and excited. But when I considered the logistics of a major move, my fluctuating health, and lack of support from family, I declined the opportunity. Instead, I diligently worked to complete the data collection on my research studies. Three years after Brennan came off treatment, I finally quit my job.

It wasn't an easy decision to give up my salary, and it was even harder to give up my professional identity. So I continued writing and publishing academic papers and mentoring my remaining students through to their final defense on my own time. But I was home after school, available every day, when Brennan bolted into the kitchen, dropped his backpack with a head-banging thump, plopped down, hoisted his monster feet up on the chair across from him, and avidly yakked about the most exciting, essential, or nagging events of his day. I savored it, steeping in the aroma of adolescent boy. I wanted the moment to last forever. His brother, meanwhile, silently slipped upstairs, retreating to his computer to escape into the medieval world of war.

I was also home when they were sick, which was once every week, according to my records. Normal kid stuff—colds, stomach virus, strep, bronchitis—but with their limited immunity to common pathogens, they just couldn't fight off the germs. And I, of course, caught everything they caught.

Once when a neighbor asked about sending her daughter over to play with Tyler, I warned her, "He has a cold."

"Oh, that's okay," she said, "she's going to get it somewhere."

I marveled at her nonchalance and envied her ability to roll with the punches of living with healthy children who were building their immune systems. And then I wondered: When her children had colds, would she tell me before I sent my son over to play? Would she understand the risk a cold virus might be to Tyler, who could easily end up on nebs and steroids for a week or two after that cold, or to Brennan, whose immune system had to start over after leukemia and whose recovery was so slow after any illness? Or to me, who caught everything and often ended up on antibiotics and prednisone myself to treat the ensuing sinus infections or bronchitis? I became paranoid, even though it would be five years before we discovered the specific immune abnormalities in all three of us that explained our susceptibility to illness.

It was exhausting staying vigilant, alert, and on top of who was sick and what virus was making the rounds. In Brennan's first year of high school, I dreamt that he had called an ambulance from home. Duane and I slept through it all. In my dream, the hospital phoned us to say that his white blood count was 300 but that he could go home.

"Home!" I screamed into the phone. "He's a leukemia survivor! Call his oncologist!" And I quickly spouted off the ten-digit clinic phone number. I remembered it in my sleep, dredged up from the deepest shades of mauve memory six years off treatment. When were we ever going to feel safe?

The dream hadn't been an irrational fear. The next morning I took one fleeting look in his throat and packed him up to head to the weekend urgent care, where the throat culture confirmed strep. My dreams had a way of alerting me.

I took on volunteer and consulting roles to stay challenged and involved in my field of research, knowing that I could work from home with just occasional travel. In some ways I was busier than ever, juggling appointments for the boys' health and my health and working around the clock when a deadline approached. The difference was, now I could work when I felt well and could also be available for the boys when I wanted or needed to be. I didn't want to have regrets. I wanted to know that I had done the best that I could, that I had thought through and anticipated what was best for my family and for me. When I got there, I wondered what had taken me so long.

CHAPTER 24

Hawaii as Refuge

When asked in second grade where he would like to go to celebrate coming off treatment, Brennan promptly replied, "Hawaii!"

Hawaii held a mystical aura for every child in the boys' elementary school. Every year the kindergarten class play-acted a trip to the islands, with the school principal piloting the airplane and the students tracking their trans–Pacific journey. Once "in Hawaii," the kids researched flora and fauna, talked story, and performed songs and hula dances for the school community.

"You've already been there!" we teased Brennan, explaining that we were in Hawaii with my sister and her family the Christmas I was pregnant with him.

Brennan, of course, was not appeased by this technicality, so, one year after coming off treatment, we hopped on a real Boeing 747 and headed to Lana'i.

The "Pineapple Island" of Lana'i no longer grows pineapples. The rich soil of the volcanic basin, where most of the 3,000 residents once worked, now grows wild with tall, grassy fields precisely lined by Cook Island pine trees. Town shops, churches, banks, and restaurants frame a one-block central grassy square, where everything Lana'i City happens. There are no commercial names, franchises, industry, or parking lots. When asked about the island, Duane always says, "There are two paved roads and no traffic lights." It's where the boys would learn to drive. It's where we took off our armor.

We were a family exploring new horizons, our boundaries not defined by cancer or illness, road maps, or schedules. My mantra on the island was "Do what we want, when we want."

Everywhere we went that week, I reconnected with my family, nature, and the universe. We drove through soft-winged ironwood trees, their arms caressing the Jeep windows on both sides and leaving a carpet of needles in the tire ruts. The forest opened to a Martian, wind-swept landscape, with iridescent purple and red sands drawing a distinct line across the horizon, interrupted only by the teetering rock sculptures standing like expressions of searching souls. A rutted, boulder-pitted road dropped straight down for miles, leading us to uninhabited shoreline where the winds whipped the sand into our legs until it hurt, reminding me who was in charge.

On the windward side of the island, we discovered centuries-old petroglyphs—warriors and animals carved into secluded boulders. We sat mesmerized in the saturating sun, watching sea turtles forage along the underwater lava rock, bobbing up and down with the swift channel surf. We were transported back in time, long before settlements, running water, electricity, and cancer.

We picnicked along the mountain ridge, with a view of three islands and fleeting glimpses of resident mouflon sheep. Closer to home, we gingerly pecked our way onto the slippery lava of the tide pools, pointing out sea cucumbers, starfish, and bright orange and black demarcated humuhumunukunukuapua'a, the state fish the boys sang about in their school songs.

On that very first trip, millions of monarch butterflies hovered around us, clinging to the purple and red bougainvillea that lined the path to the beach and lighting on our hats and backs as we walked, welcoming us in a magical rainbow of flight.

"Do monarchs migrate way over here from Mexico?" Brennan asked as he stopped to inspect one on the ground. We didn't know the answer, but it was hard to believe that so many hatched from caterpillars on the island. We would never know if this was their traditional migration path, as the following January, 80 percent of the monarch population wintering in Mexico's Oyamel fir forest died in the freezing rain. Only handfuls appear every year now.

After we returned from the trip, Brennan wrote in his journal for his third grade English class:

When I was walking from the hotel in Hawaii, I found a Monarch lying on the ground. I put it in the grass and gave it some water. When I was coming back again from the beach I checked on it and its wing had come off. I kept the wing and brought it back home. I brought it in for share. I felt like it was a friend that had died.

That was the year Max and Emily died and Kami got cancer.

Near the end of the week, we bravely skimmed fiberglass kayaks up the coastline, keeping an eye on the waves regurgitating along the thousand-foot cliffs to our right and the constant sweep of surf on our left.

"Does anyone need anything?" the young, fit guide asked us before we launched out of the harbor.

I raised my right hand high into the air. "Courage!"

"Onward!" came his reply.

When we reached Shark Fin Cove, we donned snorkel gear and jumped overboard—all except Tyler, who sat shaking in the kayak he shared with Duane. "It's too cold!" he said, shivering.

I swam over to encourage him, but I expect the rock image of the shark fin jutting out of the water was more daunting to a five-year-old. He stayed put.

We would revisit that pristine snorkeling site, by sailboat, almost every trip after that for several years, until the boys tired of the excursion. When Tyler was seven, he finally—reluctantly—put on a snorkel and jumped off the boat. After a few breast strokes through rolling waves, he popped up his head to exclaim, "This is absolutely beautiful!" Tyler's comfort level with the unfamiliar, undersea world had evolved with patience and experience, just as Brennan's resiliency with cancer had.

*   *   *

We toured a newly constructed townhome on our first trip to Lana'i in 2001, with thirty minutes to spare before a scheduled tee-time. It sat on top of a hill in the middle of the ninth fairway, right on our way to the first tee. The ocean greeted us as we swung open the heavy ipe wood door. The deep blue serenity of the ocean vista pulled us in and beckoned us through to another world. Three weeks later, we signed a contract. Three months later, we called Lana'i home.

Little would change on the island as we returned, season after season, year after year. There was security in the constancy, ritual in the consistency. Only the boys changed over the next ten years. We were redefining our world, rebuilding childhood and memories. I was grateful for every trip and every adventure together.

When the boys were ten and seven years old, I took an unpaid leave from work so the three of us could live on the island for six months, immersing ourselves in island culture and community. The timing didn't work for Duane, so he kept Minneapolis as his home base and joined us when he could.

The boys slipped easily into their fifth and second grade classrooms, eagerly keeping up with homework, adjusting to new routines, and sometimes playing with new friends after school. We often made a beeline to the beach after school, where we'd help Tyler write creative sentences with his ten spelling words each week and body surf the afternoon waves.

Later the following spring, after readjusting to life back in Minnesota, Tyler wrote for his Minnesota second grade class, "I'd like to be a turtle so that I can crawl into my shell whenever I need to." Hawaii had offered him a refuge, too.

We all gained perspective, and I'd like to believe a touch more flexibility, from changing our environment and routines and immersing ourselves in a different culture with diverse family systems. English was a second language for a third of the population on Lana'i, and many parents worked two and three jobs, leaving their children to roam through town on their own after school, adopting many "aunties" to keep an eye on them. After our six months there, I felt more synchrony with the island community, less like a visitor.

The time away was my "test drive" for eventually leaving my job. Duane had taken a new job by then and he flew out twice, once to be with the boys while I flew to Canada to give a keynote, and then to share Thanksgiving with us on the Big Island, where we paid to participate in a dolphin program I had heard about.

"But I want to swim with the *wild* dolphins," I whined afterwards. "We've been here six months!" I had watched the spinner dolphins from afar, leaping and spinning, before they either torpedoed crisply back underwater or belly-flopped as if competing for the biggest splash.

The next week the wild dolphins came obligingly into the bay while the boys were in school and I was on the beach.

Swimming with them became my passion. "The dolphins are in! Want to come?" I would yell to the boys as I burst through the door after cutting short my walk up the steep volcanic hill, from which I could spot them in the bay. Sometimes the boys would come with me, but after the novelty wore off, they declined and I got used to going alone with my snorkel gear and underwater camera. The pod of thirty-five to two hundred sometimes stayed for ten minutes and other times for four to five hours.

Seeing them swim straight at me always made me believe they had come just for me. At the last second, they would split and veer off or swim under me, some of them turning their white tummies up in a display of trust. They would always stay at least an arm's length away, and yet they seemed as curious about human behavior as we were about theirs.

One of them came to the bay several times over a year and always swam in circles around me, enticing me to follow until I sputtered into my snorkel, gasped for air, and popped up laughing. I called him Grandpa Dolphin, because he seemed all knowing and fun loving.

He once approached with two others. The three of them circled around me, tossing a piece of seaweed back and forth, nudging at each other as if competing for who could get the closest.

My most memorable moment was when one of the dolphins edged up next to me, glided parallel alongside me, and stared directly into my wide-open eyes, framed by the big clear prescription mask. I stopped moving, letting my camera dangle from around my neck, and stared back. His (or her) eye was like a huge black hole, drawing me in, sucking me into another universe. I let myself go, convinced that we were seeing directly into each other's soul.

I read every book I could find on Hawaiian spinner dolphins, thinking that if I could study their habitat, mannerisms, motivations, and ways of interacting, I would understand them better. Secretly I was also hoping to better predict when they would come into the bay, which so far I'd had no luck with. On one trip I made to Lana'i with a friend, they came every day for six days, but on other trips I didn't see them at all.

Finally, after several years of playing researcher, I realized that it wasn't about knowing more but about being there fully for the experience when they chose to be there with me. The dolphins taught me how to just "be."

One cool, cloudy day, when I ached to connect with something beyond the isolation of constant single parenting, the dolphins were nowhere to be seen. The beach was deserted. A friend from the West Coast had once suggested that I sing lullabies to them. "I can't even carry the tune of 'Happy Birthday' in the air!" I said. But that day, I hummed Joanie Bartels lullabies, warbling into my snorkel as I set out into the bay alone. Out of nowhere, a single mommy, daddy, baby triad appeared, swimming twenty feet beneath me above a backdrop of rippled sand. The parents stayed near the bottom while the baby shimmied up to me, over and over, swerving closer for a second to two and then zooming back down to glide between Mom and Dad. They led, I followed. We were the only ones in the bay for an entire hour. And then they escorted me to shallow water, the adults gave a simultaneous jerk of their head, as if to say good-bye, and they all swam off to deeper seas, baby in the middle. I sat on the beach for another hour, reflecting on the contentment, joy, and peace I felt. I was honored by their presence and their patience. I don't know what I'd satisfied in them, but they had filled an emptiness somewhere in me.

The ocean was my solace. On calm days, the waves gently lifted me up and down, rocking my soul, soothing my body, and washing away my concerns, my fears, whatever I was holding on to. One day, the current whisked away a squishy pink and yellow ball I had tucked under my swimsuit for the dolphins to play with. The force and speed of the current zipping the ball out to sea surprised me when I tossed it to a group hovering on the outskirts of the bay. After that, I often imagined my concerns being carried to the other side of the world, one ocean merging with another, like a relay passing them off, taking them far away from me. It felt good to just give them away. I sent love along those currents as well—to Kami's family, to families on the ALL listserv, to friends and family back home. I felt lighter, more buoyant in the saltwater freedom.

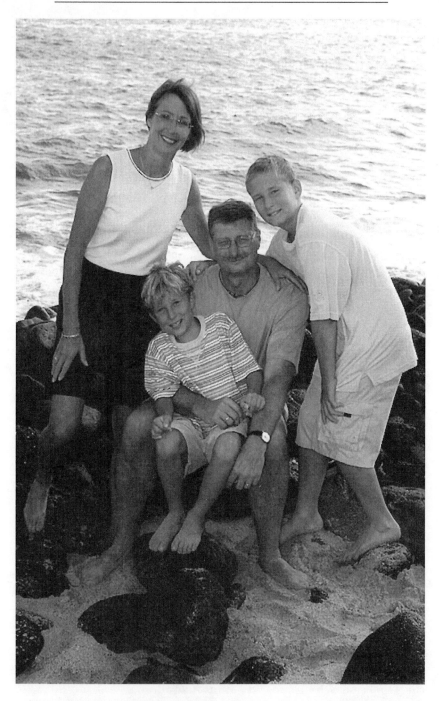

Janice, Tyler, Duane, and Brennan, Hawaii, off treatment.

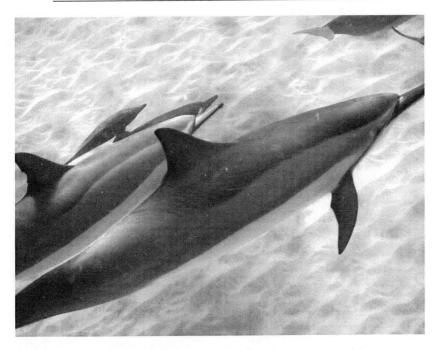

Spinner dolphins swim with the author, Hawaii.

I came alone in between family trips to retreat, reflect, and renew. Solitude was my solace. But it was our connection on our family trips that meant the most to me. The island became our place to play, to discover, and to build new traditions. We didn't plan it that way, it just happened. We had taken a risk in buying, venturing outside of our comfort zone. The adventure freed us to move on. I imagine it's like having a cabin up north on the lake, just farther away. It's a place of escape, a place to get lost in the outside world or to reconnect to the world within. Lana'i became our place to just be. On each trip, I step off the prop jet plane onto the tarmac, look up at the heavens, close my eyes, and breathe in. I am home.

CHAPTER 25

Reclaiming Childhood

Playing sports had always been Brennan's passion. After we returned from our six months in Hawaii, he eagerly jumped back into basketball, baseball, football, and golf. As he started sixth grade that fall, he announced to his oncologist that he was going to play football. He had waited for this opportunity for as long as I could remember.

"My port-a-cath is out so I can play, right?" he asked in an upbeat and expectant tone as Dr. Steve listened to his heart and lungs through his stethoscope. I was surprised that he had phrased it as a question.

"I don't see any reason why not," Dr. Steve replied in a measured voice. He glanced up at me. "How does Mom feel about it?"

His question caught me off guard. Brennan was so strong-willed and determined it would have taken his physician to veto his plan, not his mother. But given an opportunity for a say in the matter, I cocked my head and said as optimistically as I could, "It's his choice. He really wants to play." I silenced my worries. I wanted him to be free to rediscover who he was and what he was capable of, beyond cancer. I wish that I would have added, "As long as he keeps in shape."

That winter, Tyler and I shivered on the sidelines under the nighttime field lights, wrapped in thick coats and boots and sometimes with blankets tossed over our shoulders, cheering the team on as the leaves ripped from the trees in the chill autumn wind. Brennan's excitement and energy made it worthwhile. But he didn't play again until eleventh grade, by choice. And it might have been his friend who talked him into playing again. I caught snippets of banter between them as they hung out in the family room together that summer.

"We could play on the team together," Philip said excitedly.

Brennan hesitated and mumbled under his breath. Was he unsure, or was he hiding his intention from me? I could see Philip from the kitchen and his voice carried better than Brennan's, who was on the other side of the room, sprawled out on the leather couch, the one piece of furniture we had that was bigger than he was.

As I walked into the room with two berry smoothies, I heard them talking about how much weight they could lift—or, more accurately, who could lift the most weight.

"You shouldn't be bench pressing, Brennan," I said. "Not if you need someone to spot you. You can lift smaller weights and do more reps."

"That doesn't make muscle bigger," he countered, and Philip concurred by flexing his biceps.

"Yes, it does," I said, crossing my arms in front of me. "It just takes longer."

Brennan groaned. "I don't have longer."

"Isometric exercise places too much stress on your heart," I reminded him, appealing to his logical left brain but totally ignoring his teenage invincibility. Resistant isometric exercise, like pushing against a wall or blocking defense in football, would sharply increase his blood pressure and put more strain on his heart, especially if he held his breath.

The reality is that one in ten childhood cancer survivors will have heart disease by the time they are forty. The studies aren't specific to ALL, but they show childhood survivors of all types of cancer have ten times the risk of atherosclerosis and are at greater risk for arterial stiffness and valve disorders. Brennan has less risk than children who received radiation therapy to the chest (common in lymphoma) or higher doses of anthracyclines (more common in solid tumor protocols), but having a family history of heart disease, being overweight, and a lack of regular exercise dramatically increased his risk.

"I don't care," he said. But after his phys ed classes ended, so did lifting weights.

When summer came, I worried that I had squelched any motivation for exercise. Other than golf and occasional basketball and tennis, Brennan didn't move much. I couldn't get him to go on walks or bike rides anymore, and he drove a cart when he golfed with Duane. How would he be in shape to play football?

"Walking or running on the treadmill is good cardio exercise," I said one day, winking. "There's one in the basement."

"I only exercise when I have a reason to," Brennan said.

"We could bike somewhere to lunch!" I said, my pitch rising.

All I got in response was the *Come on, Mom* look.

"Well, going out for football seems like a good reason to exercise."

"I don't have to run. I'm blocking," he said and half-turned away from me.

"What?" I admitted that I didn't know the difference between a linebacker, a tight end receiver, and a defensive end. "But what about practice? Doesn't the coach make you run with the team?"

"Yeah, but I don't have to be fast." He turned and walked away.

I stopped nagging. I so wanted him to be a normal kid with childhood dreams that wouldn't just blow away in the wind.

And then another subterranean conversation between Brennan and Philip that summer put me on edge.

"I have to gain forty pounds," I overheard Brennan say.

"You need to stay in shape," I said sharply. "If you plan to gain weight, you have to exercise. You know you're at greater risk for cardiovascular disease. Besides, what about your ankles?"

He had quit playing league basketball after an ankle injury in eighth grade. Vincristine, one of the chemotherapy agents, causes foot drop in many of the kids being treated for ALL. The Achilles tendon shortens, causing tension when it contracts. Brennan's running had slowed considerably after treatment, and I noticed a flat-footed slap as he ran across the front yard, rather than a heel to toe smoothness. It slowed him down on the court, and he sometimes complained that his ankles hurt. The oncology clinic offered physical therapy, but Brennan pretended it wasn't a problem until he sprained an ankle and was out the rest of the season.

He played basketball for his high school team the following year, but this time illness benched him. Week after week, Duane and I enthusiastically climbed the bleachers after school to cheer for Brennan and his school team. Week after week, Brennan sat on the bench, cheering on his teammates. He never got on the court. After two weeks, I finally asked him about it.

"What's up, Brennan? Why don't you ever get to play?"

"I was sick this week. The coach won't let me play if I miss school anytime that week," he said in a matter-of-fact tone.

"But you've missed one day every week since school started! How realistic is that?" I clearly was less tolerant than he was. "Is it a league rule, a school rule, or the coach's rule?" He didn't answer.

"What do the other kids do when they get sick?" I asked, a little more patiently.

"Go anyway."

"They go to school sick?" I said.

"Yeah, so they can play."

"No wonder you're sick every week."

Both boys knew my stance on illness. They stayed home when they were sick, mostly so that they could rest and recover faster, but also so that they didn't spread germs. "Wash your hands!" I often reminded them. "Germs on door handles come home to all of us."

By that time I was on treatment for an immune deficiency, and both boys had been tested the previous year after they had recurring sinus infections, which are unusual in children. They both had little to no immunity to diphtheria, whooping cough, chicken pox, and pneumonia, despite vaccinations and revaccinations after chemotherapy for Brennan. Tyler had low B cell antibodies, and even though Brennan's counts appeared normal, I was sure that his natural killer cells, a specific white blood cell, weren't functioning well enough to kill germs. He caught everything, it hit him harder, and it always took him longer to recover.

He quit school basketball that season. He tired of practicing every day after school only to be benched at game time.

I tried not to play the cancer card too often, but I had joined Children's Oncology Group and was working with a team doing retrospective analyses on weight patterns for children on different ALL protocols. Many children gained weight during treatment, partly because of the oral steroids (prednisone and dexamethasone) and partly because they had little energy to exercise. The more weight they gained, the less energy they had, and the less likely they were to exercise. Most survivors never lose the excess weight, and it becomes a risk factor for diabetes, hypertension, and cardiovascular disease.

By the time football started that August, Brennan had gained forty-four pounds and Philip looked as if he hadn't gained an ounce. Sure, Brennan had grown four inches, but that weight gain was not merely height and muscle mass, despite what he said.

He cheered at meeting his goal, and his friend high-fived him. I scowled.

*   *   *

They started practicing in the mid–August heat, the day after we got home from our summer vacation in Hawaii. It was 82 degrees and hot and sticky by mid-morning. An hour into practice, one of the trainers called, reporting that Brennan had chest pain. We headed to the ER; I didn't want to take any chances with his heart.

One of the values on Brennan's echocardiogram that day had dropped 5 percent from his last test three years earlier. But the strength of his left ventricle to pump out blood was still in the normal range, even though it would decrease further on two subsequent tests. The downward trend worried me, as the effects of anthracyclines on the heart can worsen over time, but it didn't explain his symptoms that day. A combination of low sodium and potassium, dehydration, jet lag, and being out of shape were more likely explanations. He took a few days off and was back practicing the next week, until he injured his arm and spent the rest of the season advising the coach on the sidelines.

So he adapted, once again, and focused on golf, qualifying for individual state competition in his senior year. He played well on the first day and then posted his best competitive score ever on the second day. Tyler and I were spectators to his foursome. Brennan acted professional, composed, and respectful, and he sailed each drive straight down the fairway.

Just as he walked off the eighteenth green, the winds stopped dead and a sultry yellow haze rolled in with the clouds. Suddenly, the severe weather sirens blared and play was suspended.

The teenage foursomes on every hole came streaming into the clubhouse, looking around questioningly, as if to say, *The skies aren't that threatening. We've played in worse conditions.*

Tyler and I hung around the eighteenth green with Brennan and his coach, waiting for the skies to clear and play to resume. It never did. We sped home just ahead of the record fifty-two tornadoes that barreled through southern and central Minnesota that fine June day. I cautioned Brennan, who was driving the hour home alone, "Don't wait too long. Be safe!"

Brennan walked in the house just as the rains slanted their furor, propelled by forty-mile-an-hour winds.

*   *   *

The next day Brennan sat at the kitchen table with Tyler and me and read the rankings in the newspaper. The officials had used only the first-day scores to place the players. Brennan's winning score never counted. He was disappointed, as anyone would be, but he confided to us, "I played my best and that's what counts." I was sad for him, and yet I was proud of him for taking it all in stride.

At the same time, I wondered how much setback one person can accept and adapt to while still feeling a sense of hope and optimism. Brennan was still a teen discovering who he was and what he was capable of achieving.

In his senior speech that year, Brennan shared with his entire school how he never wanted to be the little engine that couldn't reach the top of the hill, the climb that the train's bigger and stronger peers wouldn't even try.

"What if the 'Little Engine That Could' never made it?" he asked himself in front of his audience. "*I think I can, I think I can, I think I can, well, I guess I can't.* That could lead to believing *I'm a failure ...* and lacking self-confidence." He continued, admitting, "I only plan things that I know have a realistic chance of succeeding."

Instead of persisting, believing, and gaining confidence with each incremental success, as the *Little Engine That Could* counsels, Brennan modified his incentive. "Never trying would be better than failing," he told his own peers. At seventeen years old, he would no longer strive to reach that crest. Instead, he would learn to be satisfied with the expectations within his reach. Or, as he often told me, "I don't make goals. Why have them if you can't keep them?"

He had lowered his expectations for himself. And yet he *had* done his best. He had persisted in playing team sports, trying one after another, and he had gone to state for golf and played well. External events had kept his score from being competitive, but he could still be proud of what he had accomplished.

I vacillated, asking how much of his perspective was that of a cancer survivor, accepting and compensating for limitations, and how much was teen boy testing out choices and asserting his values. Had he learned to accept his circumstances and make the best of what he could do because of his early life experiences? Or had his limitations squelched his motivation to keep trying? I don't know if learning compromise as a cancer survivor is a strength or a hindrance. It depended on what *his* heart felt.

* * *

In the same decade that Brennan was testing and adapting, Tyler, too, had to find his way. He was by nature an adaptable kid, one who rolled with the punches and agreeably followed along. But it was important that he find something of his own that gave him self-confidence and a sense of mastery. He played church basketball and neighborhood league baseball with the same teams for several years, making friends outside of school. He had fun, but he didn't have the same passion for sports that his brother did.

He surprised me and Duane when he asked to play hockey in third grade. "Great!" we responded, and we enthusiastically joined other hockey parents in the bleachers for chilly, all-hours-of-the-day practices. Tyler gained physical strength and stamina and he worked hard, always ready and eager for practices and games.

He played until he was eleven—and then "I don't want to play with checking," said our gentle, mild-mannered son who avoided confrontation and physical aggression.

After that, he dabbled in ceramics and art, went on bike rides and walks, hung out with friends, and volunteered at the zoo. But his real passion was forging online relationships with gamers. Most days, he retreated to his room and his virtual empires after school. He discovered who he was and what was important to him, independent of his brother.

In his senior speech, Tyler talked metaphorically of being an octopus out of water, hanging on with all eight arms in the back of a pickup truck speeding down the highway of life, as he searched for a new habitat and identity outside of his comfort zone. He had chosen to leave the ocean; it was time to move on, he told his seaworthy buddies.

We each adapted and redefined ourselves after cancer, free of schedules and road maps and constricting limitations. We made choices in a world filled with opportunities. Life felt normal.

Chapter 26

Taking On

After his first survivorship clinic visit, at the age of twelve, Brennan came home and reported to his dad with a shrug, "I had to sit through a one-hour lecture on the effects of treatment, which I just tuned out."

"What did they tell you?" Duane asked.

"I don't remember," Brennan said and went on eating.

He had a fabulous memory, but he was hearing what he didn't want to hear—"control your weight, exercise, avoid lifting weights, eat smart." I wrote the recommendations down; he ignored them.

He was an invincible pre-teen, even though he had gotten cancer. I still hoped that my mantra of "What fruit and vegetable do you want with breakfast/lunch/dinner?" would become ingrained in his subconscious. I also warned him about the risks of smoking, of course, and emphasized that drugs and alcohol make you lose control (appealing to his greatest fear). The literature reports that childhood cancer survivors tend to engage in risky behaviors less often than the average adolescent. So they do listen.

A few years later, at another annual survivorship clinic appointment, an oncologist we had never seen before asked Brennan, who was sitting across the room, "When did you come off treatment?"

"Ah, I don't know," he said, shifting in his chair.

After allowing him some time, she turned to me. "I'll bet Mom knows."

"Yes, March 6, 2000," I said quietly. But then I thought, *It doesn't matter that I remember. Brennan is seventeen; he needs to be responsible for his own health.* And that's when I became conscious of transferring the baton to him.

It was not to be an easy mission.

* * *

More children are surviving cancer today, but two-thirds of survivors of all types of childhood cancer have at least one chronic health condition (heart, lung, endocrine, or growth problems), and they are eight times more likely than their siblings to have a second severe or life-threatening illness twenty to thirty years after diagnosis. This increased risk is in part explained by their genes. As a result of treatment, ALL survivors have two hundred-fold the number of DNA mutations.

Although it's not the only factor, lifestyle can change the expression of genes at the cellular level. Brennan could start by exercising, reducing stress, and eating antioxidant-rich fruits, vegetables, and whole grains to reduce oxidation, free radicals, and telomere loss.

"You eat it because you have to," Brennan said, returning to the healthy food discussion that resurfaced over and over through the years. "I don't." *Therefore I won't,* he implied. He always needed to stake his own claim.

"Yes, but it's better for you, too," I said, a bit too emphatically.

"But it doesn't taste better."

In truth, he probably wasn't comparing organic vegetables to non-organic vegetables, but rather the choice to eat any vegetables at all. Chemotherapy had saved his life, but it had also added more oxidants and chemicals to his growing body, and the steroids had made him crave high-fat, high-calorie foods. It was a tough pattern to break after more than three years.

"Why would you spend extra money on something of no greater nutritional value?" he asked, referring to my preference to buy organic food.

That's a good question, I thought. *It means that he's considered buying organic.* "Because of the chemicals, the pesticides. Yes, I'm particularly sensitive, but so are you and Tyler, because your bodies and brains are growing."

He didn't seem convinced.

Some studies show higher levels of omega-3 fatty acids and fewer hormones in organic milk and grass-fed meat and higher levels of antioxidants, vitamin C, and phosphorous in organic fruits and vegetables. But do these differences affect health? For me, it was an issue of cumulative load and not feeling well because I couldn't metabolize the toxic byproducts from the chemicals. For Brennan, healthy eating would increase his metabolism and reduce obesity and cardiovascular disease, which are late effects of treatment. I hoped that one day he would ask himself, "Is this food good for me?" in addition to asking if it would taste good.

Two years later, when Brennan was nineteen, the nurse practitioner quizzed him instead of feeding him information and giving unsolicited advice. This was his eighth annual follow-up appointment and not much had changed, other than his weight, which had crept up the scale disproportionate to his height.

"Do you take vitamins?" she asked, her pen hovering over the clipboard on her lap.

"Nope."

"Most adults need to take some type of vitamin," she counseled, looking directly at him. "It's a good time to start."

Brennan looked down at his hands in his lap.

My mind snagged at the realization that she had referred to him as an adult. I wondered if he noticed. I expect it was intentional on her part.

"Have you had your vitamin D level checked?" she asked.

He seemed unsure, so I interjected. "Yes, three years ago. It was 34 mg/dl."

"We would like it over forty," she said.

I nodded. I would like it over fifty. But I couldn't make him take the Vitamin D3 I put out for him in the little glass dish every day he was home.

"It might help prevent some of these illnesses you've had this past year," she added, and we, the two nurses, enthusiastically nodded together. Brennan shrugged his football-sized shoulders.

"How is your vision?" she went on.

"Bad," Brennan replied, and then promptly added, "but I do fine."

"Do you wear contacts?"

"Nope."

She didn't ask if his driver's license required him to wear glasses. It did. He didn't.

"Do you wear sunglasses?"

"I don't need sunglasses," he said, reciting his typical reply. "I wear a hat."

She slipped in the word "obesity" several times. I noticed. I wondered if he did. It was a tricky topic. He didn't believe the BMI meant anything. He firmly told her, "I'm likely to die young anyway." He breathed in. "And unlike her," he pointed to me, "I oppose any preventative measures."

"But he willingly came today," I said, feeling a need to defend him or to at least give him credit for doing this for his mother. "And he had the echocardiogram."

"Yeah, if you make the appointment when I'm here, I'll come," he said, which surprised me. He had told me several times, "When I'm eighteen I am not going to any more appointments!" Now I realized he just wanted to make it clear that he had a choice.

* * *

Brennan thrived on taking the opposing stance. The summer after graduation we were sitting on the beach together when he justified to me why he refused to wear sunscreen.

"How bad is a burn on top of a burn?" he asked. I was reassured that the thought even crossed his mind. He was lying on the beach chair on his stomach because he had burned his chest playing football on the beach the day before. It was one of the few trips to Hawaii when he actually sat in the sun rather than shielding himself under a T-shirt and umbrella. I wondered if he was trying to emphasize his statement.

"I hate wearing sunscreen," he announced, as if I didn't know.

"Why is that?" I asked, playing along.

"Because I had to put it on when I was six. It doesn't matter if it's spray or lotion, scented or unscented," he went on, anticipating my comeback. "I had to wear it then, so I won't now. It's like brushing my teeth. I don't do that, either."

He once scorched his face, neck, chest, and shoulders after three hours in the water, despite many admonitions to get out and put on sunscreen. He spent the next five days inside, in pain. And even though I reminded him of that trip, he still refused sunscreen.

Childhood cancer survivors have a 4–11 percent greater risk of developing second cancers, including skin cancer, and a higher rate of cataracts from the steroids. Of course, excessive sun exposure, along with aging and genetics, increases the risk. Brennan knew this. Information wasn't going to change his behavior.

"Does your red-headed, fair-skinned girlfriend wear sunscreen?" I asked, leaning into peer pressure.

"Oh yeah. Just like the rest of the world." And then he got up to cool off in the surf. Sans sunscreen.

*　*　*

I had to trust that eventually Brennan would take on more initiative for his health. For someone who needed control, he was slow to take responsibility. Although I suppose *not* taking responsibility is perhaps a way to control.

As a member of Children's Oncology Group, I witnessed the consequences of cancer treatment at every meeting. The teams of physicians, nurses, and other clinicians and scientists continually strove to increase survival rates and improve outcomes and quality of life for survivors. Once they saved the children, they wanted them to live well.

As we waited for a session on cancer epidemiology to start at one fall meeting, several colleagues—mothers and fathers of healthy pre-teens and teenagers—animatedly compared notes on what their kids were doing or not doing with their lives.

"My son just went off to his first year of college," a renowned statistician proudly announced.

"What about your older son?" I asked, remembering that his oldest and Brennan were about the same age. "What is he up to now?"

"Oh, his mother kicked him out of the house last winter. He quit college and was home, lying around on the couch trying to decide what to do with his life. He would still be there if she hadn't shown him the door."

I was shocked. These were bright, talented, and *healthy* kids of high-achieving parents. What had gone wrong? Brennan had hugged the couch and preferred solitude and darkness between the ages of thirteen and fifteen. After those two years, he suddenly resurfaced, rejoining family life as if nothing were amiss. But the stakes seemed higher as they got older.

It impressed me that these parents had enforced a consequence. It's easy for kids to shirk responsibility if they aren't held accountable, even if the parents couch it as "We only want what's best for you." I was taking notes; Brennan had been talking about dropping out of school. As first-generation college graduates from lower-middle class families, both Duane and I strongly valued education, so of course we opposed this idea.

I sat down as the session began, feeling ambivalent about these kids, especially the boys, who seemed to need more time to mature, find out who they were, and decide on their life's path. And then it dawned on me: This was typical teen behavior! Seeking and mulling over and even avoiding responsibility was a developmental stage.

This didn't excuse Brennan's behavior, of course, but suddenly I realized that my son was very much like other young men his age. He was alive! He was normal! I breathed a huge sigh of relief and turned back to the speaker, who was talking about neurocognitive effects of intrathecal chemotherapy. I came home from that meeting thankful for my son's life and very, very grateful for having these developmental struggles to face. I had to believe that he would find his way.

Just two weeks later we drove the five hundred miles to Brennan's college for a football game. After listening for years to Brennan dispute the value of a chemical-free, organic diet, I gloated, without saying a word, when I opened his refrigerator in his first apartment and spotted organic eggs, milk, broccoli, and strawberries, and filtered water.

"The organic carrots really do taste better," he said with a straight face.

CHAPTER 27

It's Okay to Cry

My father taught me how to face my fears. In death, he showed me how to let go.

My father's journey paralleled Brennan's passage from preschool to high school graduation. His heart attack, four months before Brennan's diagnosis of leukemia, left him with 50 percent of his heart cells but 100 percent of fight. Over the next thirteen years, through Brennan's elementary, middle school, and high school years, my father managed his ensuing congestive heart failure by taking a handful of new medications and exercising faithfully. In between two lung cancer surgeries, spaced ten years apart, he miraculously survived blood clots that originated in his heart and migrated to his abdomen and legs—though not, thankfully, to his brain. By comparison, Brennan's road map felt far more predictable.

Despite his repeated medical crises, my father didn't talk about death unless it was in the past tense—as in, how he had dodged it. I don't know which he feared more, death itself or dying alone. Or maybe he just loved life too much to leave it. He had been an amateur, competitive ski jumper and golfer, and he had continued golfing into his 80s, adapting his swing after his first thoracotomy.

After his heart attack, twenty-four hours after we had flown home from Disney World together, a friend told him, "If you had had that heart attack on the plane, you would be dead." Dad refused to fly again.

I watched him endure inconceivable pain and suffering over and over as he repeatedly fought off death. And every time I asked him in a crisis, "Where do you want to be, Dad?" he always said, "Right here"—in the hospital. I don't know if that's because he felt more hope or safety. Or both.

He bargained for yet another chance during Brennan's senior year of high school. As my parents and I sat on cold metal chairs in the surgical conference room that snowy January day, waiting for the surgeon, my father told me how it felt before he was "shocked back to life" after his heart attack, thirteen years earlier.

"It was quiet, peaceful, with no pain, no noise," he said.

I looked up at his prominent German nose and watched his translucent blue eyes fill with tears.

"It will be the same, you know," I said to him quietly.

He nodded.

It was the first time we had given voice to death. I saw him hesitate. He wasn't ready to let go just yet. And it was a good thing, because he was scheduled for his second lung cancer surgery within the week. He needed to want to live.

I wanted to ask him if he was alone when he was brought back to life, or if anyone was there to greet him, but the surgeon walked in just then.

Before the doctor even had a chance to sit down, my father said abruptly, "I want you to know that if my heart stops on the operating room table, I don't want you to restart it. I've been through that before. They shocked me six times with my first heart attack. Once was enough." He took a quick breath and added, "I've had thirteen extra years, and for that I'm grateful."

I actually thought I heard him hoping he could slip away that easily.

The surgeon—a tall man with delicate hands, rounded fingertips, and a gentle nature—slowly and calmly looked into my father's eyes and replied, "We like to bring our patients back out of the operating room when we take them in." And that was the end of the conversation.

My father survived the surgery, but it wasn't curative this time. A month later, when he was finally home from the hospital, he called me at home at nine in the morning. The early hour told me it was important.

"I just wanted to tell you that I'm not sure I want to do anything more," he said to me. "I don't want to suffer any more. I've lived eighty-two years. That's long enough. I'm ready to die." As if expecting a rebuttal, he said, "I know what's best for me, and I'm going to stand up to the doctor on Tuesday. I'm not afraid. They aren't going to do anything without my okay."

He needed to talk out his thoughts and hear me validate his decision. I was thankful that he felt comfortable sharing them with me. Just the day before, he and my mother had said, "We will do whatever the doctor tells us to," and I had backed down from my mantra of "You do have a choice. You always have a choice."

I gently told him as we said our good-byes over the phone, "I will support you in whatever decision you make, Dad. I will be with you every step of the way."

Sharing our suffering, feeling connection and compassion, helps us feel a little less alone. In the process of voicing our fears we come to accept them, releasing their hold on us. Sharing was my father's first lesson in letting go.

*　*　*

We started Brennan's senior year knowing that it likely would be my father's last. Dad had avoided death for thirteen years, and I knew better than to have any expectations. I did, however, have hopes and dreams for Brennan.

As I walked into my last back-to-school night for high school parents, I thought back to Brennan's first day of kindergarten, when he stood tall and proud in his white collared shirt and navy blue pants, smiling outside of his classroom door. He seemed like every other enthusiastic five-year-old starting school.

And then images of school, coinciding with his first year of cancer treatment, slithered out from my subconscious. Most days, I followed him into the school building, one step behind him as he tilted his whole body back and yanked with his long, thin arms to open the two heavy oak school doors. His gait quickened as he walked down the hall and to the stairs, always smiling as he slipped through the open kindergarten door, cheerfully greeting his new friends and confidently sitting down at a table to do a puzzle or play a game. At noon, after recess, we exited through the same secure doors and, half an hour later, walked through the easy-to-open door to the oncology clinic, the one with a window and a clear view into his other world of shots and leukemia treatment. He worked so hard to be strong and successful in both worlds.

And here we were, twelve years later, survivors, anticipating graduation and a life beyond the shelter of school and any cancer credentials.

Over the years, the school had accepted, nurtured, and challenged Brennan—and, most important, allowed him to be who he was. At seventeen years old, he strategically considered his options, confidently defended his beliefs, took responsibility for his choices (even when they diverged from mine), and consistently supported the underdog. He knew how it felt to face the odds. I wondered how I would ever make it through graduation day with such a whirlpool of emotions.

* * *

My father began to prepare us for his passing. He often began his sentences with "If I don't make it through this [current crisis]" or ended his statements with "I have to die of something, honey." I never knew if he was preparing himself or me.

His strength and resolve became even more apparent in his final weeks. After an emergency admission to the cardiac care unit, he made the decision to stop taking his heart meds. He knew the consequences. His determination convinced all of us that this truly was his wish. And yet he had to remind his medical team of this three times as he transferred from the cardiac care unit to the oncology unit and then, lastly, to the extended care facility. Either communication was ineffective or each new team was testing him, wanting him to be sure.

"I'm not taking those pills anymore," he reminded the nurse. "You need to take the medications for my heart off my list." He wasn't angry, although he looked up at me with tight lips as if to ask, "Why can't they get this right?"

When I visited, early evening became our time alone. The hospital floor was quiet, no one interrupted, and the winter sun set early, casting a drowsy darkness, illuminated only by the yellow glow of a lamp behind the curtain. It reminded me of Dad sitting in his knobby, upholstered chair in the living room, reading the newspaper after dinner under the glow of the ancient, bronze floor lamp.

On our first evening alone, we talked about the Saturdays he'd taught the four of us kids how to downhill ski and ice skate. We reminisced about our summer excursions fishing off shore with a bamboo pole and climbing pine trees like monkeys when we got bored watching the red and white bobber sitting too still on the water. When I leaned over him to kiss him goodnight, tears poured unannounced down both of our cheeks. He met my gaze, his clear blue eyes gentle and caring behind pools of tears, and whispered his first lesson to me: "Remember the good times, honey."

I nodded, biting my quivering lip. Yes, I could do that.

When Dad was settled in the extended care center, I had to decide about our family's last spring break trip to Hawaii. Was I being selfish to want to escape with my family for this one last trip before Brennan headed off to college? This would be the last time our boys would have two weeks for spring break and the last time their spring breaks would coincide.

My three siblings were all coming to visit my parents while I was gone. They would be there for Mom's eightieth birthday and for Dad. And they would have each other. This was all rationalization, of course, a cover for my real fear. *Will I be able to live with my guilt if he dies while I'm in Hawaii?*

My father knew I was struggling with the decision and yet he let me make it, even though it broke my heart to have to choose. One night during our time alone, he said in a firm voice, "Don't feel guilty, honey. I know what it's like to have a family. You do what you need to do." I wouldn't realize until years later that in my effort to make the right decision for *me* I had forgotten just how important it was to *him* to have all of his family together. Jerry had been missing from my father's last Christmas, and now I was missing from his final family time. Not feeling guilty has been one of the toughest lessons my father taught me.

In the end, we went to Hawaii. It was hard to be so far away, and yet we had some of our best talks over the phone while I was there. I called him from the beach every night at the usual time we would have been alone together. I wasn't with him to clean his teeth or give him a backrub or help him get ready for bed, but he knew I was with him in spirit.

"Are the dolphins in?" he asked one day.

"Yes, they are leaping and twirling just sixty yards from shore," I said, always calculating distances as if I were about to make a chip shot.

"And are Duane and Brennan on the golf course?"

"Yes! You knew, didn't you?"

And then later, at the end of our twenty-or-so-minute conversation, he said, "You go chase those dolphins now, honey."

It might have been his signal to end the conversation, as my mother said later, but to me it was more than that. I was surprised that he could track and remember the details of our conversation so clearly, despite the hefty doses of pain meds he was on. And I was honored that as his strength dwindled, at a time when most people turned inward, he was thinking of me and my passion. Every time I sit on the beach and watch the dolphins now, I think of my father's strength and compassion and his lesson in valuing and honoring play.

✳ ✳ ✳

Despite his fear of dying alone, Dad believed, and probably wished, that his heart would fail at night while he slept.

Ultimately, it did.

It was Easter week, early Wednesday evening, as I sat next to his bed facing him, the blinds of the big picture window open at the head of his bed. A full moon gently ballooned over the horizon, blazing a deep golden orange and shadowing the still bare branches of the maple trees. I described it to him, my eyes fixed on the scene as if willing the moon to protect him.

"The moon is huge, Dad. It's right outside your window, beaming in." I paused, feeling warm energy flow through me. "You know, Dad, the courage in your heart is like the full moon growing bigger over the horizon, rising bravely into the sky."

Several days later, when I told my mother about the moon, she told me that the full moon had always meant something special to my father. She never said "emotional," she just said "meaningful." "Maundy Thursday was important to him too," she said.

Maundy Thursday is the day Christians honor Jesus's death on the cross. It's also the day my father took his last breath.

I turned to look at my father, noticing how sallow and drawn his face was. His mouth was open wide, taking in and releasing slow, shallow breaths. His temperature had risen to 102 degrees that afternoon. I planned—and needed—to drive the two hours home that night because I was scheduled for an intravenous infusion of my immune therapy the following day. Surprisingly, I didn't feel pressure or angst, just an incredible sense of knowing and peace. The words poured from my heart, from a place buried deep beneath decades of family silence and denial surrounding death.

"Dad!" I said, exclaiming in surprise at my sudden awareness, my discovery. "The reason your heart is so strong is because it is filled with so much love." I envisioned his heart pumping out eighty-three years of love and passion for living. "And so much determination and courage," I added, thinking about the thirteen and a half years since his heart attack. And, knowing it played a huge part in his survival, "and a sprinkling of German stubbornness tossed in." If he could have smiled, I expect he would have. I placed my right hand on the center of his chest, leaned in so I was inches from his face and said softly and slowly, "We feel your love, we know your determination, and we honor your courage. These are your gifts to us. We will carry them with us. It's okay to let go of them when you are ready."

I left him at 7 p.m., the end of our usual time together, with Selah's "You Raise Me Up" playing in the CD player next to his bed. I wasn't there at 2:35 a.m. My family wasn't there. And the nurse apologized that she wasn't with him when he took his last breath. But I don't believe he died alone.

At about 4 a.m., I was talking out loud to my father, telling him how relieved I was that he had finally found peace, and I suddenly heard the refrain "Joy, joy, joy, joy." It echoed in my head, over and over again, for an hour. I walked around my house smiling. I was absolutely convinced that Dad was with me, telling me that he was free, free of pain and worry. It was then that I realized that he wanted us to celebrate his life with joy. After all, he was joyous.

* * *

After Dad's memorial service, as I sat at the cemetery underneath the black tarp shielding his family from pouring cold rain, I heard him say his last lesson to me: "It's okay to cry, honey." But I couldn't then. The sky was doing the crying for me.

As my father shepherded me through his death, he gave me a gift for living. In facing his own fear with strength and courage, he showed me how to face mine. In acknowledging his own vulnerability, his humanness, he allowed me to begin to unlock my emotions, the feelings I had buried since childhood. He allowed me my choices, and honored my needs, at a time when his were so great. He was with me every step of the way.

* * *

I flew out to Hawaii three weeks after my father's funeral, on my annual solitary retreat, honoring the time to process his death and to feel his spirit outdoors in nature, a backdrop for which we shared a fervent passion.

It was Allison's death that reminded me to be grateful for every day.

I had been in Lana'i only a few days when I received a late-night e-mail from the boys' school. Allison, one of Brennan's ninety-four classmates, had died that day. I reread the e-mail again, my face pressed close to my phone.

It was after midnight back home. I immediately texted Brennan. "What happened? Had she been sick? Did you know?" I fired away, hoping he was still awake. I couldn't wait until morning for answers.

"Yes, yes, and yes," he replied promptly.

"Tell me more," I pleaded on screen, waiting inches away for a response, imagining him lying back in his bed, his head propped up on pillows, his computer on his lap and his phone in his hand.

"She didn't come to school on Monday. She apparently had a stroke Sunday night."

I sat transfixed on the floor. Why hadn't he told me? I had talked with him almost every day that week. He and Allison had sung in their choir concert together on Saturday night. We had seen her less than a week ago. I ached to be home with him, to talk to him, to share his grief (even though he didn't let on to owning any), and to share mine. Once again, I straddled the continents, literally and figuratively. I felt left out, alone, searching for answers and insight, something that would make sense to me and console me. I had come to Hawaii to escape my daily routines and give myself time and space to process my own grief, and yet I hungered to be there for my son as he faced yet another death at school. Allison was the second of Brennan's classmates to die and the fourth child at the school to die since Brennan had started kindergarten.

I felt drugged by death. I sat cross-legged on my bedroom floor, 4,000 miles away, reading and rereading the black words swirling on the white screen. I wanted to know Allison better. I wanted to know her likes and dislikes, her personality, her goals in life. I wanted to feel her presence. I have no idea why I needed or wanted to feel closer to more loss, more grief, four weeks after my father's passing. I felt myself gliding down the slick slide of sorrow; I saw the bottom beckoning. *"It isn't fair!"* I wanted to scream. But I stayed silent, rocking back and forth ever so slightly, my hands clutching my cell phone.

The suddenness and unexpectedness of Allison's death heightened my sense of vulnerability. Life, again, felt so incredibly fragile. Just when I was starting to feel safe again, helplessness and grief surged up, overtaking my confidence. It could have been us. It could have been Brennan.

For years I had believed, trusted, that we were doing everything we could to ensure our son's survival, prevent relapse, and reduce the late effects that could compromise health and longevity. But my expectations of control vaporized the day Allison died. I knew then that despite all of my efforts, death could happen to any child, to any family, to any one of us, at any time. I had watched Max and Kami and Caelhan die of cancer. I had seen their families suffer and endure the deepest pain a parent can ever know. But Allison had been healthy. There had been no time to prepare, to say good-byes. Safety was an enigma, control an illusion. Allison's death taught me that there are no certainties in life, only hopes and dreams and infinite doses of trust and faith to move us forward.

I stayed in Hawaii for two weeks, observing events through Brennan's lens. Back at home, the energy at his school moved like sludge. Final exams for seniors were canceled, sports games forfeited. I quizzed Brennan on every detail.

"What are students doing?" I asked one day when we talked on the phone.

"Sitting around in the commons, talking, hugging, crying."

"What are you doing?"

"Mostly practicing for the memorial service."

The choir, who had sung together with Allison at Carnegie Hall a year before and at their spring finale just two weeks earlier, joined voices one last time to sing "Let It Be" at her memorial service.

When I talked to him later that evening, he said the church had been packed and lots of people had stood up to share stories of Allison. He answered my questions dutifully, but his voice sounded flat, drained. I could feel the heaviness through the phone line slowing my own thoughts and reactions. I had no antidote to grief.

"So, what now?" I asked, wondering if it was too soon to be "moving on" so quickly but wanting to offer a glimmer of anticipation, of hope. Graduation was just a month away. It was supposed to be a happy time, a time of anticipation and celebrations, of hope for their future.

"We will start our internships Monday."

As planned, I noted. We talked about his upcoming internship as a sports broadcaster with the Twins. I was thankful he had something to look forward to.

* * *

I flew back across the ocean the next day, ready to inch forward, step by step, consciously aware that ninety-three sets of senior parents, me included, would be preparing to live without their child for a semester, while Allison's parents would go on living without their daughter forever. I imagined her family organizing her pictures in a collage from birth to death while I created a slideshow of Brennan's life, choreographing pictures and video clips to his favorite music. There were so many pictures of him with my father—Dad hoisting him up to the basketball hoop, showing him how to swing a golf club, playing mini golf and real golf with him, pitching him the plastic "baseball" in the yard, and playing Schmier with everyone at every family get together. I oohed and cried and laughed and sighed through the entire marathon weekend. It was a surprise gift, and in the end, the DVD seemed more meaningful to me than to Brennan. His childhood had been my gift, after all.

As Brennan prepared to graduate and move on, I tried to focus on the good times, let go of my regrets, and allow myself to cry and play. I would have to face my fears or I would carry those buried emotions with me forever. I wanted love, not fear, to infuse my life.

CHAPTER 28

Letting Go

Graduation was held outdoors on the school lawn, freshly cleansed by a midday June rain. Arriving early, we chose third-row seats on the farthest side so I could take pictures without blocking someone else's view.

My father's absence was palpable. He had always been the photographer at family events—the one to set up the tripod, click the timer, and run into place, usually next to Mom. He had been present for every important event in the boys' lives—births, baptisms, all of their birthdays, and even some of their school events. When Tyler was in third grade and my father had just come home from the hospital, he and my mother drove ninety miles to attend Tyler's "Spotlight On," a day their school highlighted one student with a poster, mementos, and family/class interaction. My parents had been there for Brennan, and they wanted to be there for Tyler, even though my father could barely walk the block from the car to the school.

It had been a hectic five days leading up to graduation, with senior prom, Brennan's eighteenth birthday, choir and graduation practice, and parties. I was running on adrenaline, rushing from one event to the next, coordinating logistics and photographing milestones. My father had teased Brennan at Christmas that Tyler would get his driver's license first. When he was admitted into the hospital that winter, I told Brennan, "I can't be here to drive you to golf when I need to be in Wisconsin with Grandpa." At the same time I confided to my friends, "He likes having a chauffeur, chef, and concierge." And I really didn't mind being those things for him. I realized, however, that I was enabling his dependence—and, undoubtedly, clinging a bit too tightly to his childhood. By graduation, I was thankful my older son could drive himself.

I sat down dutifully as *The Graduation March* began. The girls, in white dresses, and the boys, in navy blue blazers and white pants, paired up to walk through the ivy trellis, treading cautiously on the wet, tarp-covered grass. I smiled at their poise and confidence as a suite of emotions rushed through me, guided by the orchestra of sweet flutes, booming tubas, and rhythmic drums.

When the choir sang "For Good," a song from the play *Wicked*, I was so close I could distinguish Brennan's strong tenor voice, convincing me that the lyrics of how others shape who we become were meant as much for me as for his classmates and teachers. I watched my son's mouth shape every word with heart. I felt joy and pride, brush-stroked with relief. I silently thanked Brennan's strength and resilience for getting us through three years of cancer treatment and for helping him find his way as a survivor. For the entire day, and even the rest of the month, it was easy to ignore the emptiness looming ahead.

✻ ✻ ✻

Two weeks later, after his state golf tournament, Brennan and I flew out to Hawaii to have a week alone together before Duane and Tyler and then Brennan's three friends joined us. It was the first time we had gone on a trip with just the two of us.

We lay side by side on beach chairs, watching the waves glisten in the midday sun, listening to the breaking surf rush up the white, powdery sand and then retreat, snapping and crackling along the shoreline rocks. I soaked up that rare moment, breathing in the connectedness I felt to both my son and the ocean's rejuvenating energy. He was doing this for me, and I was grateful.

"Why do you like the beach so much, Mom?" he asked, as he had off and on over the years.

"Someday you might appreciate the sitting and doing nothing," I replied as I kept my gaze on the sparkling ripples.

In anticipation of the trip, I had jotted down a list of questions, hoping to find out more about who my son was as a person now that he was going off on his own. Sitting on the beach gave us a rare opportunity to talk without multitasking or doing. I wanted to ask, "What motivates you, energizes you? What makes you feel good about yourself? What gives you confidence? What helps you when life feels chaotic? What makes you happy?" But I didn't ask these questions. Was it because I didn't want to feel as if I was interrogating him? Or was it because I still handled emotions like glass that could shatter? We had focused on survival for so long, avoiding such deep questions, that I wasn't sure he would be receptive to them.

One of the questions I did ask was "What is it that you want?"

"I just want to be happy," Brennan said in earnest, turning to me and shielding his eyes from the sun. "I don't want to be one of those people who admit later in life, 'Why did I do all that? Why did I sacrifice my happiness just to be successful?'"

His seriousness prompted my own introspection. "I want you to be happy, too," I said sincerely, my mind searching for who he might be taking his cues from, who his role models were. Would he consider his father successful but unhappy? It was hard to decipher emotions with Duane. Somewhere along the way, I suspect that he, too, had learned to hide, or suppress, or deny them. After all, what you hide from others you hide from yourself.

In the ensuing silence I added, "You have to discover what makes you happy," respecting that his values could differ from mine but also implying that I didn't expect him to already know. What I wanted to convey was that true happiness comes from within. But I think he already believed that.

"I don't expect to live a long life," he said pensively.

I always tensed when he said this, but after hearing it a few times, I had deduced that it was his way of valuing short-term happiness over long-term survival. He was making it clear—again—that he didn't want to take care of himself "just for that payoff." This was his vista as an adolescent edging into adulthood.

"The important thing is that it is a conscious decision, a choice you are making," I said. I was trying so hard to love and listen, not to solve and resolve. His health and happiness were now his responsibility. I had to allow him that in order to let him go.

"Yeah. At some point it might change, but that's what I want now."

"I can't really look beyond the next three days," he said.

"That seems like it might be a typical attitude of any college student."

"I make my decisions by weighing the risks and rewards and doing what seems right at the time. My actions are based on who I am and not on what society expects of me."

"Or what your parents expect," I added. He didn't always make the best choices, but he always had a logical rationale for his actions and accepted the consequences that followed them.

At age fourteen, Brennan had refused to go to confirmation the second year because he just couldn't "buy into the business aspect of church." I coaxed and coerced, but he was too big to drag into the car. One day, as I drove his friends home from tennis, he said in response to some predicament or decision he had confronted, "So I added God to my list [of appeals], just in case there was one listening." He saw it as covering his bases; I saw it as a glimmer of realization that life might be bigger than just him.

Expectations and grades were equally unimportant to him, even when his GPA determined college acceptance. He would only invest time and energy if it was something he wanted. He didn't want to get a college degree just because society expected, valued, and rewarded education. It had to be right for him.

As I sat, nodding in contemplation, mesmerized by the sparkling horizon and my son's unwavering beliefs, he added, "I want to live authentically."

My eyebrows went up; I was surprised by his comprehension of what for some is an elusive concept. How was it that I was just learning to live true to my own self, to stop carrying water for everyone else, when he was already figuring out as a teenager what he needed to do to honor who he was and who he wanted to be?

I didn't ask him what he thought "living authentically" meant. I couldn't second-guess that kind of knowing. Next to me was a young man who had endured three years of invasive, sickness-generating, prescribed treatments just to survive his childhood. And here he was, a decade later, announcing his courage to live his life fearlessly in the moment, seeking happiness and embracing who he was and what he believed in. He'd already grasped this enormous task that many of us strive our entire life to achieve. I could see my father's strength, courage, and determination in my just-turned-eighteen-year-old son. What goal could be more defining than that?

*   *   *

August arrived and college move-in day loomed. "I'll pack later," Brennan kept saying—which, when you live in the moment, means "the morning of."

After an eight-hour drive and two days of hauling and shopping and setting up a bed, television, and refrigerator—the typical college move-in routine—we commanded him away from his new roommate to come say good-bye to us, his former roommates of eighteen years.

I gave him a hug; he let me. I think he actually hugged me back, sort of. The kind of hug a ready-to-move-on eighteen-year-old boy gives his mother. I looked up into his eyes—gray-blue, like mine—as they peered down from almost a foot above me. Only three years earlier, we'd looked straight into each other's eyes when we stood face to face.

"Text me—or call me," I said. "I'll want to know how you are doing." Checking in and talking to him every day was what I would most miss. I wondered if he, too, would miss our after-school check-ins and late-night explorations of things we found stimulating or vexing.

Brennan briefly nodded and turned away, and I caught a fleeting glimpse of shiny armor. Perhaps it reflected a bit off my own.

After a last parental montage of "Good-bye, be safe, and have fun," Brennan turned and walked back down the narrow, dark hallway to his room on the left, second from the end. It was after noon on a gray, cloudy day, and the north-facing window at the end of the hall let in just enough light to illuminate his six-and-a-half-foot frame, dressed in black and white athletic shorts and topped with a Tigers hat. I watched him saunter off to his future, the one that he planned. I smiled with relief, confidence, and a vacuum of emptiness.

Duane commented as we pulled out of the parking lot, "I'm surprised Mom isn't crying."

"Maybe it hasn't sunk in yet."

* * *

I cried every night for a week after we got home. The house was *so* empty without Brennan's energy. I missed hearing his deep, strong voice with its confident opinions and commanding presence, questioning my every action with "Why would you do that?" My heart pleaded into the darkness, *Why do you have to leave me just as I am getting to know you? You know, though, don't you, how very much I love you?*

Which made me question if he did know. Had he known that I loved him even when I reassured him instead of really listening to his concerns or acknowledging his emotions? Did he know I loved him when I witnessed facts instead of feelings, when I searched for answers instead of asking the right questions? Could he see that it was my love for him that powered my pleas to take care of his body?

Of course, it was me who needed to forgive myself. I had buried my regrets for years, acknowledging them only when they surfaced in my dreams. Guilt and regrets aren't all bad. They motivate us to change, to do better next time. But dwelling on the past can get us stuck. It was time to move on. I had to learn *from* them, not learn to live *with* them. I practiced forgiving myself in the shower every day.

* * *

Six weeks after dropping Brennan off at college, during one of our almost weekly conversations, I mentioned that I should start cleaning his room. "I haven't done much except wash the clothes that were on the floor."

"I don't care what you do with my bedroom; I don't live there anymore," Brennan said.

My breath caught in my chest as I quickly tried to think of the right thing to say. I measured the words out in a careful monotone. "I like to think you will feel at home in your bedroom when you do come, even if it's just for a visit." I exhaled slowly. I was proud of myself for not blurting out what I really felt: *What? Of course you will! This is your home forever!*

It would take me weeks to get the courage to sort and clean out his room and closets. He had given me permission to "do whatever you want with whatever is left." Being a minimalist, he had taken very little with him. *Did he purposely leave all these memories for me to face alone?* I wondered with every item I uncovered, tears flowing readily down my cheeks. I carefully selected and tucked away the mementos from his coming-off-treatment party, his eighth birthday, his "Light the Night" T-shirt from the Leukemia and Lymphoma Society survivor walk we did with my sister and niece in St. Louis, and the pictures of him half a lap ahead at the American Cancer Society Relay for Life. *See how far you've come,* they seemed to say. I tried to accept his absence by walking back through the years.

For months, I peered out at the empty space on the street, directly in view of my second-floor office window, where his car had come and gone at all hours. The familiar rectangular black imprint on the street was now covered in fallen leaves. I had stayed awake every night that summer before college, waiting for his car to pull up, to know that he was safe at home. I smiled at the number of nights that dragged on to three and four in the morning, when I was so ready for him to go off to college so I could get some sleep. I still sometimes find myself waking up at 3 a.m. and peering out the window, expecting—wishing—his black SUV will pull up in the dark of night.

And that's when I miss him the most: when the house is quiet and the television is off and his bed is made. I still crave his energy, his intensity, his questioning of everything mundane to philosophical, his ability to take over a room, his bigness. When it gets too quiet I replay all those irresolvable questions he posed throughout the years.

"If you knew it was your last meal, what would you eat?"

"If you had a time machine, would you go back in time or forward in time? Why?"

"Why do we have an English language?"

"Why do people practice a particular religion? Any religion?"

"How can anyone be 'right' about what's 'right' and 'wrong'?"

And then the questions became more abstract. Questions like how *The Matrix,* string theory, chaos theory, and quantum mechanics explain the world. I never understood the questions, much less the answers. I could, however, understand that everything relates to everything else, and our actions and even our thoughts have repercussions in our body and in other matter, even reaching into other planes of existence, in a nonlinear and unpredictable way. I imagine that's how grief and loss reverberate through the cells of our body and may even reach out and touch others energetically. Having studied immune and neurohormone signaling between the mind and the body, I got that our biology, and even our genes, respond to our beliefs. Our minds are the matrix of matter.

I could even conceptualize how the string, or the wave, or the fluttering of a butterfly's wings initiates an energy ripple, causing a much greater effect at a distance. Like the ocean waves rolling gently out at sea, blips easily paddled in the canoe, they build height and momentum until they come crashing down on shore. It takes experience and patience to land a smooth exit in a canoe. I learned that it's not about predicting the waves, or even avoiding them, but flowing with and riding them in. Unless it's a tsunami; then I'd run.

We couldn't run from leukemia. A twang on Brennan's string triggered a response in all of us. We learned to ride the waves, each with our individual goals for survival and getting through. While I faced the waves head on, Tyler ducked under them and escaped, as best he could. And although Duane often withdrew to the comfort of the shore, preferring negotiation and discussion after the intensity calmed, he was there for back-up. Ultimately, we were on the same boat, constantly balancing and navigating. We landed safely, changed but intact.

The dynamics in our house changed after Brennan left, but the string still seemed in his control. Now that we no longer needed to slay the dragon, our challenge was to reprogram our responses, from stress and reactivity to intention and thoughtful appraisal. I began to open to a new rhythm of receiving in exchange for the energy of giving. I felt less need to parent and more need to simply connect.

Adapting is a process. When Brennan comes home, it's like a big wave whooshing me back in time, all the expectations tumbled with joy. And then he leaves again, and the sand settles on the deserted beach. I savor the moments, trusting that the emptiness will ebb over time, just as it must for all parents. Letting go is my path to peace, but it sure is a tumultuous ride.

CHAPTER 29

Shadows of the Heart

Hawaii, December 2011

I was dreaming.

The doorbell rang.

I answered it.

Brennan had died.

In my dream, my son's teenage friends walked through the door, one by one. I couldn't look at them. Arms without faces handed me a horse, a dog, a basketball, a football. All stuffed. All white. All memories. I didn't want them. I didn't accept them. But I took them. With each one, I turned and walked the few steps to the white painted ledge of the dining room bay window. The window seat was barren, white, and cold. The corner of my eye glimpsed a lone, large bouquet of vibrant flowers, centered on the table in the midst of nothingness, suspended like a rainbow after a storm. I wasn't ready to see color.

My hands, like robots, dropped each gift, one on top of the other, as my head turned away. My heart thumped, ready to run away if it could. I turned my back on the growing pile. Objects could never fill the emptiness mounting inside of me, a black balloon expanding in my chest. The balloon might explode. I needed to live in the darkness, to feel it, to be it. I turned back to take the next gift, as if the rhythm of moving back and forth would keep me alive.

"He needs to be here for Tyler," I insisted to the bodies without faces that never said a word. "I need him here," I implored, as if begging him to do this one last thing for his mother. The silence informed me. He wasn't going to be there for his brother's high

229

school graduation. He wasn't going to be there for me. Not then, not ever again.

* * *

When I awoke, fear replaced grief.

It was 2:40 a.m. The same time my father had died. I was alone in our island home. I had never feared being alone, but now the blackness gripped me. It obliterated everything except the red numbers on the clock. Only my thoughts moved.

It had been eleven years since Brennan had completed treatment for leukemia. For the first time in my dreams, my son had died. I had no idea what the circumstances of his death were. It didn't seem to matter. It was the ominous void that haunted me. For the first time I could remember, I felt helpless. I couldn't save him.

There were no tears in the dream. Crying might have made things messy, uncontrollable. Over the days that followed, my heart pulsed with unknowing and uncertainty, along with a new awareness, a seeping vulnerability. He was safe! Why couldn't I let go? Why were my fears coming back to haunt me, when denying them had once protected me?

Tears flowed afterwards, day after day, as I walked up the 20 percent-grade climb by my home, a place where red hot lava had once descended, tumbling over the sheer cliff, lighting the night sky with a story that only history could tell. Tears overflowed with every memory, allowing some tiny release from the volcanic pressure of sorrow and fear that had collected inside me over the years.

The dream taunted me for two weeks. I had come alone to our island retreat to reflect and to write. But the feelings were too intense; words never reached the page. One evening I climbed the hill to watch the sun settle over the ocean. The sky softened in pinks and blues, like blankets draping babies' cribs. The clouds gently transformed, dotting the sky with cotton ball fluff. And there, lying in a cloud, was my son, his nineteen-year-old body nestled in a coffin. All white and still, amidst a changing sky. I stared, stone still, holding my breath. For a few long moments we both were transfixed in space. I forced my breath in and out, wishing his chest to rise and fall with mine.

Were the dream and the clouds an omen? Was Brennan going to die?

Do I dare admit that my subconscious mind was toying with fears that had flamed for years, licking at the memories of my son's vulnerability through three years of treatment for leukemia? He was a survivor. And yet I remained hypervigilant. It was as if the memories had weaseled their way into my cells, lurking in my DNA, regenerating insidiously. Wasn't it time to lay these fears to rest? If only I could understand them, make sense of them, see them materialize into words on paper—maybe then, I thought, I could let them go.

* * *

Brennan's tonsillectomy was scheduled for early January, within days of the fifteenth anniversary of his diagnosis. The day of his surgery, back in Minnesota, I sat alone in the muted surgical waiting room and stared at the black heart painted in the abstract picture hanging on the wall. Fears blurred into one. Memories flooded back, a torrent of tears catching up with time.

A tonsillectomy was routine, but as a nurse I knew that every surgery carries risk. The adult son of one of my colleagues died after he had his wisdom teeth removed, and Brennan had experienced reactions to anesthesia in the past. Even he admitted in the car on Christmas Day as we drove home from the movie *Les Misérables*, "I *could* die." Was that what I too was thinking as I sat shaking, suppressing sobs, as we sat side by side in the theater listening to Jean Valjean pine for injured Marius as he sang "Bring Him Home"? Still, as Brennan emphasized the "could," he shooed away the probability. Statistics were his passion and he would place his bet on the odds. It was harder for me. We had already faced that slim probability, the unfathomable chance of childhood cancer.

I didn't worry during daylight hours. I was confident of Brennan's cure from leukemia. But when he died in my dream one month before his tonsillectomy, fear rang the doorbell with a clarity I couldn't deny. He had died in my dream. And I had answered the door, allowing my subconscious entrance to my fears.

Fear isn't logical or rational. Fear is waking in the night drenched with sweat or shivering with cold. Fear grips and doesn't let go. It invents the worst that can happen and then smolders through the day, licking away at energy, confidence, and faith, leaving ashes in its footsteps. When events sort themselves out, as they usually do, fear retreats and we go on our way, none the wiser. Unless we turn back and ask fear what we can learn from it.

Forgetting doesn't heal; remembering does.

* * *

Three hours after Brennan's tonsillectomy, which took place across the street from Children's Hospital, in the hospital for adults, we drove the well-worn path home in the car. This time, Brennan sat in the front passenger seat, squashed into the bucket seat of my little sedan. He held a cold pack to his neck.

"So, what's for dinner?" he asked, as if it were just any errand we were running together.

I turned to him, a questioning look in my eyes.

He questioned me back with his.

He was serious about eating. Three hours after surgery on his throat, the path to his stomach was ready to get on with life.

I turned back to the road, laughing joyously. "Whatever you want," I told him. And I smiled the biggest smile my heart could hold.

Epilogue

As seems to be the case with all of life's lessons, I had more opportunities to practice what I had learned from my son's leukemia. In 2014, two years after Brennan's tonsillectomy, when he was back at college and getting sick much less often, my twin brother died suddenly and unexpectedly. Jerry was fifty-eight years old and the first of my siblings to die, leaving a mother to outlive her son.

"No, not Jerry!" I wailed into the phone to my younger brother, expecting the midday call to be about our mother's well-being. Our brother's death defied logical order; it assaulted our expectations. Once again I was face to face with death, my fears, my own vulnerability, and the question "What am I supposed to learn from this?"

It took me weeks to realize I had lost not only a brother but a twin, a soul entwined with mine. On Friday night, three days before his death, I'd said to my mother over the phone, "Jerry's Christmas cactus is drooping." He had sent us the plant as a housewarming gift exactly thirty years earlier, to the month. "It's bloomed every year, sometimes twice a year. I wonder if I'm overwatering it," I said to Mom, who understood plant maladies much better than me. She knew plants, I knew bodies—or so I thought.

The glossy green succulent had sat next to me in my home office for years, growing bushy and bursting forth with cheerful red blooms right on holiday cue, keeping me company on my writing journey. And then it suddenly lost vitality. Just like my brother.

And then I lost mine. On Monday morning, while he lay on his office floor at the university 2,000 miles away, paramedics slicing through his steel gray biking shirt and attempting to resuscitate him, I unknowingly sat in my kitchen immobilized, lethargic, void of energy or explanation, wondering why I felt so drained. It would be four hours before I had my answer.

Jerry had always been the strong one, the athletic one. He was the twin who had gone home from the hospital first, the healthy one, the one who from day one had challenged his body almost as rigorously as his mind. I was the second, smaller twin, a surprise to our parents. Isolated alone in the hospital after birth, I fought to survive, to overcome. Over the years, when friends and acquaintances asked if my twin had health issues too, I always replied, "No, he got the good genes." How wrong I was.

"Focal, severe coronary arteriosclerosis," the autopsy report read. "Left main coronary artery ninety percent blocked." There was minimal atherosclerosis and no disease, no malady, anywhere else in his body. Jerry was as focused in death as he was in life.

"All the men in my family died young of heart disease," my mother blurted out within minutes of my arrival at her house that heartbreakingly clear and temperate Monday afternoon.

I stared at her as she stood unsteadily in the middle of her dining room, her voice distraught, projecting the truths silenced through the years. I took in this new awareness. "Really?"

At that point we had no cause of death, we just assumed it was his heart. Why hadn't we thought of our mother's side of the family when Jerry said he had trouble breathing four minutes into biking, running, and swimming? Was it because he had gone on to ride another fifty-four miles just two days before he died? Or because we all expected to live into our nineties as our paternal grandparents, the side of the family we knew about, had?

Why is it so hard to see the evidence laid out in front of us when it is our loved ones that hurt? I had missed the cues in my father, my son, and now my brother. Was it that I couldn't be objective or that I didn't even want to go there? I'm too responsible to blame destiny.

It had taken me years to process and release the guilt of not seeing my father's impending heart attack and not recognizing cancer in my son's symptoms. And now a new trigger, and the same response. Guilt. The burden of responsibility, of expectations for myself, sat like a resolute brick on my chest. We certainly couldn't ignore death now.

I drove back from my mother's before sunrise and boarded the plane to meet my younger brother at the coroner's office and do what had to be done. It was how I knew to "get through," to survive. I set aside the processing, the making sense of it all, as I had with my son's diagnosis, and I focused on the tasks at hand.

When we couldn't find a will, and couldn't break the code to get into his computer, I leaned against the wall in Jerry's upstairs room—a space scattered with electronics, the place in his house where I most felt his presence—and asked him aloud where to find it. Within minutes I had a manila envelope labeled in his scratchy handwriting, just like mine, "Will, May 2012," in my hand. I had found it lying flat on top of the box of tax returns, the only paper documents he owned. I had searched in that closet, even moved that box, hours before. All I needed to do was to ask and to listen. And then my eyes could see.

On the plane ride back home, when I couldn't "do" any more in the moment, guilt careened back without warning. We had taken care of Jerry's house and finances and canceled his appointments and four upcoming flights. We had gone every day to the university where he taught, filing papers and sharing stories with the dean, faculty, and students. But on that last day, the finality of seeing, and then leaving, my brother's body in preparation for its final trip back to Wisconsin sank into my seat with me.

"His death was totally preventable," I spewed out heatedly as I hurriedly stowed my bag and plopped down next to my seatmate, a slim, retired pediatrician on his way home from a fly fishing trip to Canada. We had both been serendipitously assigned to new seats at the last minute.

"Maybe not," he replied kindly, gently.

Those two simple words and his calm certainty settled me into my seat. "Maybe not," I said to myself, over and over. We sat in silence as I absorbed his permission to let go of the guilt once more. And then he listened as I shared my brother's passion for biking, exercise, and adventure, and I relayed the symptoms leading up to his sudden death. By this time, five days later, all I could think of was how classic his symptoms were and how we, including two physicians he had gone to that summer, had all missed the ominous signs of heart disease.

"I'm kind of like your brother in my passion for adventure and athletics," the retired doctor said as he turned toward me halfway into the flight. I so appreciated how he talked to my eyes and not to the wall in front of us. "The only thing I could do differently"—he paused, looking directly at me—"is to be female ... and stay young."

He let the idea of having no control sink in. He seemed okay with it, which made me feel as if I should too. And then we talked the entire way home, as the cabin darkened and quietness settled around us, about the risks we take and the choices we make—about life, about death, about living.

Thank you, I whisper over and over as the months creep by. *Thank you for your grace, your gentleness, and your caring enough to correct my destructive thinking.* I see how holding on to guilt serves no purpose once the lesson is learned. Regrets are inevitable. They inspire us to do better next time—to be strong but also to accept our own weakness, uncertainty, and not knowing.

I trusted this man's knowledge as a physician, but it was his humanness that granted me peace. Instead of burying my emotions and masking my insecurities, as I had all those years after Brennan's diagnosis, I felt them—and, more important, in the throes of my raw, uncensored, and fresh grief, I shared them. In doing so, I gained clarity and peace. A compassionate soul had listened to my grief and my guilt and had helped me to move on, to accept my limitations, my humanness, without expectation.

Back in Minnesota, exactly one week after Jerry's death, I returned from my walk and spotted a bright yellow Stella D'Oro daylily in the midst of dried, crunchy leaves. It was 27 degrees outside and everything else had frozen or gone dormant for the season. As I focused the camera to take a picture of this one brilliance in my morning, I saw a second flower closely attached on the same stem. It was shriveled and small, withering alongside the yellow flower. I realized that I, not my twin, was meant to be the bright yellow surviving flower. I sat down on a rock and sobbed.

The next day after my walk, there were two more flowers, both of them a brilliant yellow, blooming side by side on the same stem, looking in the same direction. According to Taoist tradition, a yellow flower, especially with its petals projecting outward, is the highest stage of enlightenment, an absence of desire and suffering. I knew then that my twin walked beside me.

I continue to focus on the good times, but only those in the past, because when I yearn for the future, my loss is unfathomable. Jerry had been looking to buy a vacation home in Hawaii. It was where we had planned to play together. After a divorce and decades of teaching, he was finally going to play.

"He always wanted a house on the beach," Jerry's friend John told me. So, six weeks after his death, we built him a sand castle on the beach in the bay. We sat for hours under the umbrella telling Jerry stories, watching the tide flow gently in and smooth away the turrets.

"John, look!" I cried out as I walked closer to inspect the new shape, molded by the incoming tide, that sat on top of the entrance next to the yellow hibiscus flower we had placed there.

"It's a Chinese lion," said John, a practitioner of Chinese medicine. "He's guarding Jerry's castle."

"Yes!" I said, and then mused to myself, *And he's sending us strength and courage.*

Acknowledgments

Many thanks to Elena Ladas, trusted and talented coauthor, colleague, and friend, who sparked the flame for this book with her enthusiasm and confidence. And to my dear friends and colleagues—Anne Hannahan, who started me on the path forward, and Katherine Brown-Saltzman and Susan Bauer-Wu, who supported me with their loving presence and our cherished writing retreats through my son's treatment and all the years beyond.

In deep appreciation to Janet Jones, who knew just when to encourage and when to step back, but always gently blowing on the flames. And when I most needed confidence, Mary Rockcastle emerged with encouraging feedback and a shared connection to our past.

A heartfelt shout-out to fellow childhood cancer parent and writer Stacy Prince, who over the years shared stories, memories, and anxieties, along with hopes and dreams for our children and our books. I am honored to be the recipient of her boundless encouragement and steadfast friendship.

I am grateful for the years of Terran Lovewave's patient coaching to let go, watch and observe, and learn to "be" and not "do."

I am indebted to the visionary creators, mentors, and teachers of the Loft Literary Center of Minneapolis and to Elizabeth Jarrett Andrew, my first memoir mentor, who so patiently guided me, step by carefully thought-out step, through the process and discovery of craft and story. My deepest thanks go to my dedicated writing group: Rebecca Molloy, Nicole McKenzie, Karli Lundberg, Beth Kodluboy, Char Miller, Lisa Kee, and Heather Dewar Langner, and my other memoir mentors: Cheri Register, Brooke Warner, and Linda Joy

Myers, for their insightful and critical feedback as my story and skills unfolded. With your perpetual help, I eventually found cohesion and clarity. And to Susan Kilby and the attentive and patient team at McFarland and Toplight Books, thank you for sending my story out into the world.

Thank you to my family for letting me tell my story. For Brennan, in honor of your courage, bravery, and fight for your life, and your respect of my beliefs. I do this for you. For my husband, Duane, for being there, allowing me my need to take charge, and honoring the unspoken silence—for years, which is how long it took for me to sort out my own thoughts first. And to my son, Tyler, who cared enough to ask what creative nonfiction was in his first year of college, for honoring my closed door sequestering, and for his unwavering smiles, hugs, *I love you's*, and way too many *Happy Birthdays*!

In honor and in memory of my father, Vernon O. Post, who modeled courage and compassion when facing fear, and my twin brother, Gerald (Jerry) V. Post, who bravely did everything first and showed me how to be the best I could be. Thank you to my mother, Doris, my sister, Elaine, and my brother, Ted, and his wife, Cathy, for being there for me throughout our journey.

My heartfelt appreciation to Sara Froyen Gernbacher and to all the nurses who shared in our story as parents and children navigating the cancer world. In gratitude to Drs. Stephen Nelson and Susan Sencer and the Hematology-Oncology team at Children's Hospital and Clinics, who were steadfast and meticulous clinicians and leaders in their field—and who, most importantly, harbored no assumptions and were patient with me, a new cancer mom.

A special thanks to Laurie Larson, Dr. Beth Frankman, and Christopher Priebe for rescuing me so many times and for your ongoing love, support, and commitment to our family. And although these words will never reach Nancy Bone and Sarah Gutknecht, I hope you knew how very much Brennan and I appreciated your dedicated presence in the clinic and hospital as we inched along through three years of treatment.

Blessings and peace to the families of Max, Kami, Caelhan, Allison, and Emily, who have only their memories to hold on to. My heart breaks for you. And yet I witnessed your incredible strength in enduring.

And to all the families traveling their own journeys, whose stories are as meaningful as mine: Be strong, be brave, but allow yourself to be human.

Bibliography

Chapter 4

Ford, Anthony M., Chiara Palmi, Clara Bueno, Dengli Hong, Penny Cardus, Deborah Knight, Giovanni Cazzaniga, Tariq Enver, and Mel Greaves. "The TEL-AML1 Leukemia Fusion Gene Dysregulates the TGF-Beta Pathway in Early B Lineage Progenitor Cells." *The Journal of Clinical Investigation* 119, no. 4 (2009): 826–836. https://doi.org/10.1172/JCI36428.

Hübner S., G. Cazzaniga, T. Flohr, V.H. van der Velden, M. Konrad, U. Pötschger, G. Basso, *et al.* "High incidence and unique features of antigen receptor gene rearrangements in TEL-AML1-positive leukemias." *Leukemia* 18, no. 1 (2004): 84–91. https://www.nature.com/articles/2403182.

Shurtleff, Sheila, Arjan Buijs, Fred G. Behm, Jeffrey E. Rubnitz, SC Raimondi, ML Hancock, Godfrey C.F. Chan, C. H. Pui, Gerard Grosveld, and James R. Downing. "TEL/AML1 Fusion Resulting from a Cryptic t(12;21) is the Most Common Genetic Lesion in Pediatric ALL and Defines a Subgroup of Patients with an Excellent Prognosis." *Leukemia* 9, no. 12 (1995): 1985–1989. https://pubmed.ncbi.nlm.nih.gov/8609706/.

Zelent, Arthur, Mel Greaves, and Tariq Enver. "Role of the TEL-AML1 fusion gene in the molecular pathogenesis of childhood acute lymphoblastic leukaemia." *Oncogene* 23 (2004): 4275–4283. https://doi.org/10.1038/sj.onc.1207672.

Chapter 5

Binder, Elisabeth B., and Charles B. Nemeroff. "The CRF System, Stress, Depression and Anxiety—Insights from Human Genetic Studies." *Molecular Psychiatry* 15, no. 6 (2010): 574–588. https://doi.org/10.1038/mp.2009.141.

Bowlby, John. *Attachment.* New York: Basic Books, 1982.

Gotlib, Ian H., J. LeMoult, N.L. Colich, L.C. Foland-Ross, J. Hallmayer, J. Joormann, J. Lin, and O.M. Wolkowitz. "Telomere Length and Cortisol Reactivity in Children of Depressed Mothers." *Molecular Psychiatry* 20 (2015): 615–620. https://doi.org/10.1038/mp.2014.119.

McGowan, Patrick O., and Moshe Szyf. "The Epigenetics of Social Adversity in Early Life: Implications for Mental Health Outcomes." *Neurobiology of Disease* 39, no. 1 (2010): 66–72. https://doi.org/10.1016/j.nbd.2009.12.026.

Szyf, Moshe. "The Early Life Environment and the Epigenome." *Biochemistry and Biophysics Acta* 1790, no. 9 (2009): 878–85. https://doi.org/10.1016/j.bbagen.2009.01.009.

Wolynn, Mark. *It Didn't Start with You: How Inherited Family Trauma Shapes Who We Are and How to End the Cycle.* New York: Viking Press, 2016.

Chapter 6

Angström-Brannström, Charlotte, and Astrid Norberg. "Children Undergoing Cancer Treatment Describe Their Experiences of Comfort in Interviews and Drawings." *Journal of Pediatric Oncology Nursing* 31, no. 3 (2014): 135–146. https://doi.org/10.1177/1043454214521693.

Chapter 7

Moore, Thomas. *Dark Nights of the Soul: A Guide to Finding Your Way Through Life's Ordeals.* New York: Gotham Books. 2004.

Chapter 9

"Causes of Leukemia: Bibliography of Journal Articles." *Ped-Onc Resource Center.* Last modified January 11, 2018. http://www.ped-onc.org/diseases/leukcauses biblio.html.

Falak, Riza, Mojtaba Sankian, and Riza Varasteh. "The Possible Role of Organophosphorus Pesticides in Augmentation of Food Allergenicity: A Putative Hypothesis." *Research Journal of Environmental Toxicology.* 2012. 6: 88–100. https://doi.org/10.3923/rjet.2012.88.100.

Gouveia-Vigeant, Tami, and Joel Tickner. "Toxic Chemicals and Childhood Cancer: A Review of the Evidence." *University of Massachusetts Lowell Center for Sustainable Production, University of Massachusetts Lowell.* 2003. Accessed December 26, 2020. http://www.sustainableproduction.org/downloads/Child%20Canc%20Exec%20Summary.pdf.

Lawson, Christine C., Carissa M. Rocheleau, Elizabeth A. Whelan, Eileen M. Lividoti Hibert EN, Barbara Grajewski, Donn, Spiegelman, and Janet W. Rich-Edwards. "Occupational Exposures Among Nurses and Risk of Spontaneous Abortion." *American Journal of Obstetrics and Gynecology* 206, no. 4 (2012): 327.e1–327.e8. http://www.ncbi.nlm.nih.gov/pmc/articles/PMC4572732/.

Newcombe, David S., Ali M. Saboori, and Ahmed H. Esa. "Chronic Organophosphorus Exposure: Biomarkers in the Detection of Immune Dysfunction and the Development of Lymphomas (abstract)." *ChemInform* 25, no. 21, 1994. https://doi.org/10.1002/chin.199421312.

"Possible Environmental Causes of Childhood Leukemia." *Ped-Onc Resource Center.* Last modified January 11, 2018. http://www.ped-onc.org/diseases/leukcauses.html.

Rea, William J., and Hsueh-Chia Liang, M.D. "Effects of Pesticides on the Immune System." *Journal of Nutritional Medicine* 2, no. 4 (1991): 399–410. Accessed December 26, 2020. http://informahealthcare.com/doi/abs/10.3109/13590 849109084143.

Zahm, Shelia Hoar, and Aaron Blair. "Pesticides and Non-Hodgkin's Lymphoma." *Cancer Research* 52, suppl 19 (1992): 5485s-5488s. https://pubmed.ncbi.nlm.nih.gov/1394159/.

Chapter 10

Krull, Kevin R. "Neuroanatomical Abnormalities Related to Dexamethasone Exposure in Survivors of Childhood Acute Lymphoblastic Leukemia." *Pediatric Blood & Cancer* (2019) e28118. https://doi.org/10.1002/pbc.28118.

Walsh, Catherine P., Linda J. Ewing, Jennifer L. Cleary, Alina D. Vaisleib, Chelsea H. Farrell, Aidan G.C. Wright, Katarina Gray, and Anna L. Marsland. "Development of glucocorticoid resistance over one year among mothers of children newly diagnosed with cancer." *Brain, Behavior, and Immunity* 69 (2018): 367–373. https://doi.org//10.1016/j.bbi.2017.12.011.

Chapter 12

Daskalakis, Nikolaos P., Edo Ronald De Kloet, Rachel Yehuda, Dolores Malaspina, and Thorsten M. Kranz. "Early Life Stress Effects on Glucocorticoid—BDNF Interplay in the Hippocampus." *Frontiers of Molecular Neuroscience* 68, no. 8 (2015). https://doi.org/10.3389/fnmol.2015.00068.
The Institute for Functional Medicine. "Genome-Wide Changes May Result from Excessive Stress." *Insights, The Institute for Functional Medicine.* Accessed December 28, 2020. https://www.ifm.org/news-insights/gene-genome-wide-changes-may-result-from-excessive-stress.
Luebbe, Aaron M., L. Christian Elledge, Elizabeth J. Kiel, and Laura Stopplebein. "In Children with Psychiatric Disorders, Higher Cortisol was Associated with Greater Behavioral Outbursts and Lack of Self-Regulation." *Journal of Clinical Child and Adolescent Psychology* 41, no. 2 (2012): 227–38. https://doi.org/10.10 80/15374416.2012.652000.
Pöder, Ulrika, Gustaf Ljungman, and Louise von Essen. "Posttraumatic Stress Disorder Among Parents of Children on Cancer Treatment: A Longitudinal Study." *Psycho-Oncology* 17 (2008): 430–437. https://doi.org/10.1002/pon.1263.
Reynolds, Rebecca M. "Glucocorticoid Excess and the Developmental Origins of Disease: Two Decades of Testing the Hypothesis." *Psychoneuroendocrinology* 38, no. 1 (2013): 1–11. https://doi.org/10.1016/j.psyneuen.2012.08.012.
Rosenberg, Abby R., Joanne Wolfe, Miranda C. Bradford, Michele L. Shaffer, Joyce P. Yi-Frazier, Randall Curtis, Karen L. Syrjala, and K. Scott Baker. "Resilience and Psychosocial Outcomes in Parents of Children with Cancer." *Pediatric Blood and Cancer* 61 (2014): 552–557. https://doi.org/10.1002/pbc.24854.
Unternaehrer, Eva, and Gunther Meinlschmidt. "Psychosocial Stress and DNA Methylation." In *Epigenetics and Neuroendocrinology*, edited by D. Spengler and E. Binder, 227–261. Switzerland: Springer International Publishing, 2016. https://doi.org/10.1007/978-3-319-29901-3_1.

Chapter 16

Stoneham, Sara, Lynne Lennard, Pietro Coen, John Lilleyman, and Vaskar Saha. "Veno-Occlusive Disease in Patients Receiving Thiopurines During Maintenance Therapy for Childhood Acute Lymphoblastic Leukaemia." *British Journal of Haematology* 123, no. 1 (2003): 100–102. https://doi.org/10.1046/j.1365-2141.2003.04578.x.
Stork, Linda C., Yousif Matloub, Emmett Broxson, Mei La, Rochelle Yanofsky, Harland Sather, Ray Hutchinson, *et al.* "Oral 6-Mercaptopurine Versus Oral 6-Thioguanine and Veno-Occlusive Disease in Children with Standard-Risk Acute Lymphoblastic Leukemia: Report of the Children's Oncology Group CCG-1952 Clinical Trial." *Blood* 115, no. 14 (2010): 2740–2748. https://doi.org/10.1182/blood-2009-07-230656.

Chapter 17

Sulkers, Esther, Wim JE Tissing, Aeltsje Brinnksma, Petrie F. Roodbol, Willem A. Kamps, Roy E. Stewart, Robbert Sanderman, and Joke Fleer. "Providing Care to a Child with Cancer: A Longitudinal Study on the Course, Predictors, and Impact of Caregiving Stress During the First Year after Diagnosis." *Psycho-Oncology* 24 (2015): 318–324. https://doi.org/10.1002/pon.3652.

Chapter 18

Greeff, Abraham Petrus, Alfons Vansteenwegen, and Annelies Geldhof. "Resilience in families with a child with cancer." *Pediatric Hematology Oncology*.31, no. 7 (2014): 670–9. https://doi.org/10.3109/08880018.2014.905666.

Grootenhuis, Martha A., Bob F. Last, Johanna H. De Graaf-Nijkerk, and Monique Van Der Wel. "Secondary Control Strategies Used by Parents of Children with Cancer." *Psycho-Oncology* 5 (1996): 91–102. https://doi.org/10.1002/(SICI)1099–1611(199606)5:2%3C91::AID-PON212%3E3.0.CO;2-N.

McCubbin, Marilyn, Karla Balling, Peggy Possin, Sharon Frierdich, and Barbara Byrne. "Family Relations: Family Resiliency in Childhood Cancer." *National Council on Family Relations* 51, no. 2 (2002): 103–111. https://doi.org/10.1111/j.1741–3729.2002.00103.x.

Patterson, Joan M., Kristen E. Holm, and James G. Gurney. "The Impact of Childhood Cancer on the Family: A Qualitative Analysis of Strains, Resources, and Coping Behaviors." *Psycho-Oncology* 13 (2004): 390–407. https://doi.org/10.1002/pon.761.

Rosenberg, Abby R., Joanne Wolfe, Miranda C. Bradford, Michele L. Shaffer, Joyce P. Yi-Frazier, J. Randall Curtis, Karen L. Syrjala, and K. Scott Baker. "Resilience and Psychosocial Outcomes in Parents of Children with Cancer." *Pediatric Blood and Cancer* 61 (2014): 552–557. https://doi.org/10.1002/pbc.24854.

Chapter 19

Kadan-Lottick, Nina S., Pim Brouwers, David Breiger, Thomas Kaleita, James Dziura, Veronika Lu Chen, Megan Nicoletti, Bruce Bostrom, Linda Stork, and Joseph P. Neglia. "Comparison of Neurocognitive Functioning in Children Previously Randomly Assigned to Intrathecal Methotrexate Compared with Triple Intrathecal Therapy for the Treatment of Childhood Acute Lymphoblastic Leukemia." *Journal of Clinical Oncology* 27, no. 35 (2009): 5986–5992. https://doi.org/10.1200/JCO.2009.23.5408.

Matloub, Yousif, Susan Lindemulder, Paul S. Gaynon, Harland Sather, Mei La, Emmett Broxson, Rochelle Yanofsky, *et al.* "Intrathecal Triple Therapy Decreases Central Nervous System Relapse but Fails to Improve Event-Free Survival When Compared with Intrathecal Methotrexate: Results of the Children's Cancer Group (CCG) 1952 Study for Standard-Risk Acute Lymphoblastic Leukemia, Reported by the Children's Oncology Group." *Blood* 108, no. 4 (2006): 1165–73. https://doi.org/10.1182/blood-2005–12–011809.

Chapter 20

Buchbinder, David, Jacqueline Casillas, Kevin R. Krull, Pam Goodman, Wendy Leisenring, Christopher Recklitis, Melissa A. Alderfer, *et al.* "Psychological Outcomes of Siblings of Cancer Survivors: A Report from the Childhood

Cancer Survivor Study." *Psycho-Oncology* 20, no. 12 (2011): 1259–1268. https://doi.org/10.1002/pon.1848.

Long, Kristin A., and Anna L. Marsland. "Family Adjustment to Childhood Cancer: A Systematic Review." *Clinical Child and Family Psychology Review* 14, no. 1 (2011): 57–88. https://doi.org/10.1007/s10567–010–0082-z.

Tarr, Jill, and Rita H. Pickler. "Becoming a Cancer Patient: A Study of Families of Children with Acute Lymphocytic Leukemia." *Journal of Pediatric Oncology Nursing* 16, no. 1 (1999): 44–50. https://doi.org/10.1016/S1043–4542(99)90006–1.

Chapter 22

Bozarth, Alla Renee. *Life Is Goodbye Life Is Hello: Grieving Well Through All Kinds of Loss.* Minnesota: Hazelden Foundation, 1994.

Chapter 25

American Heart Association. "Childhood cancer survivors at elevated risk of heart disease." ScienceDaily, 26 August 2019. www.sciencedaily.com/releases/2019/08/190826092316.htm.

Gibson, Todd M., Matthew J. Ehrhardt, and Kirsten K. Ness. "Obesity and Metabolic Syndrome among Adult Survivors of Childhood Leukemia." *Current Treatment Options in Oncology* 17, no. 4 (2016): https://doi.org/10.1007/s11864–016–0393–5. nihms769663.pdf.

Jarvela, Liisa S., Harri Niinikoski, Olli J. Heinonen, and M. Paivi. "Endothelial Function in Long-Term Survivors of Childhood Acute Lymphoblastic Leukemia: Effects of a Home-Based Exercise Program." *Pediatric Blood and Cancer* 60 (2013): 1546–1551. https://doi.org/10.1002/bc.24565.

Piper, Watty. *The Little Engine That Could.* New York: Grosset and Dunlap, 1990.

Rosen, Galit P., Hoai-Trinh Nguyen, and Gabriel Q. Shaibi. "Metabolic Syndrome in Pediatric Cancer Survivors: A Mechanistic Review." *Pediatric Blood and Cancer* 60 (2013): 1922–1928. https://doi.org/10.1002/pbc.24703.

Zhang, Fang Fang, Shanshan Liu, Mei Chung, and Michael J. Kelly. "Growth Patterns During and After Treatment in Patients with Pediatric ALL: A Meta-Analysis." *Pediatric Blood and Cancer* 62 (2015):1452–1460. https://doi.org/10.1002/pbc.25519.

Chapter 26

Armenian, Saro H., Wendy Landier, Melissa M. Hudson, Leslie L. Robison, Smita Bhatia, on behalf of the COG Survivorship and Outcomes Committee. "Children's Oncology Group's 2013 Blueprint for Research: Survivorship and Outcomes." *Pediatric Blood and Cancer* 60 (2013): 1063–1068. https://doi.org/10.1002/pbc.24422.

Blackburn, Elizabeth, and Elissa Eppel. *The Telomere Effect: A Revolutionary Approach to Living Younger, Healthier, Longer.* New York: Grand Central Publishing, 2017.

Byrne, Jennifer. "Cure for Childhood Cancer May Come at the Cost of Premature Aging." *HemOnc Today,* February 10, 2020. Cure for childhood cancer may come at the cost of premature aging (healio.com).

The Childhood Cancer Survivor Research Study—Publications. *St. Jude Children's Research Hospital.* 2020. Accessed December 28, 2020. https://ccss.stjude.org/published-research/publications.html.

Chow, Eric J., Kayla L. Stratton, Wendy M. Leisenring, Kevin C. Oeffinger, Charles A. Sklar, Sarah S. Donaldson, Jill P. Ginsberg, *et al.* "Pregnancy After Chemotherapy in Male and Female Survivors of Childhood Cancer Treated Between 1970 and 1999: A Report from the Childhood Cancer Survivor Study Cohort." *Lancet Oncology* 17, no. 5 (2016): 567–76. https://doi.org/10.1016/S1470-2045(16)00086-3.

Gordijn, Maartje S., Raphaele R. van Litsenburg, Reinoud J. Gemke, Marc B. Bierings, Peter M. Hoogerbrugge, Peter M. van de Ven, Cobi J. Heijnen, and Gertjan J. Kaspers. "Hypothalamic-Pituitary-Adrenal Axis Function in Survivors of Childhood Acute Lymphoblastic Leukemia and Healthy Controls." *Psychoneuroendocrinology* 37, no. 9 (2012): 1448–56. https://doi.org/10.1016/j.psyneuen.2012.01.014.

"Late Effects of Treatment for Childhood Cancer (PDQ®)—Health Professional Version." *National Institutes of Health, National Cancer Institute.* Last modified December 4, 2020. https://www.cancer.gov/types/childhood-cancers/late-effects-hp-pdq.

"Late Effects of Treatment for Childhood Cancer (PDQ®) Patient Version." *National Institutes of Health, National Cancer Institute.* Last modified March 10, 2020. https://www.cancer.gov/types/childhood-cancers/late-effects-pdq.

"Long-Term Follow-Up Guidelines for Survivors of Childhood, Adolescent, and Young Adult Cancers." *Children's Oncology Group.* Version 5 (2018). Accessed December 28, 2020. Guidelines.indd (survivorshipguidelines.org)

Index

Numbers in *bold italics* indicate pages with illustrations